'This extraordinary, edited volume is ba  first conference of its kind exploring the writings of C. G. Jung and Gilles Deleu expertise offered here provides a much· of rhizomatic holism found in Jung and Deleuze, out is ... expanded to assist readers in realizing the tremendous implications for 21st-century psychology and philosophy. The editors are to be celebrated for crafting this remarkable collection; it will not disappoint!'

Joseph Cambray, PhD, President/CEO,
Pacifica Graduate Institute, USA

'The configuration of systems and the relationships of interconnecting parts to a whole is a fascinating conceptual puzzle, and one vital to our understanding of the functioning of society and our relationship with ourselves, others, and the world at large. *Jung, Deleuze, and the Problematic Whole* asks important epistemological and ethical questions of wholeness through the lens of heavyweight thinkers, Gilles Deleuze and C. G. Jung. Written by experts in continental philosophy and Jungian studies, this book is insightful in its scrutiny of a variety of interrelated issues, including reductionism, totalitarianism, privilege and exclusion, identity, creativity, and personal and social transformation. A wholly compelling book.'

Lucy Huskinson, Professor of Philosophy,
Bangor University, UK; author of *Architecture and
the Mimetic Self*

'*Jung, Deleuze, and the Problematic Whole* is essential reading for those interested in the flourishing area of Jung/Deleuze studies. From a Jungian perspective, Deleuze's ideas allow an interpretation of Jung's writing on the *unus mundus* that both critiques and revitalizes his work. For those who study Deleuze, this is added evidence of the potential for a psychology consonant with the ideas of schizoanalysis. Overall, this book marks an important contribution to the ongoing exploration of Jung's influence on the philosopher of the rhizome.'

Barbara Jenkins, Professor, Department of Communication
Studies, Wilfred Laurier University, Canada; author of *Eros and
Economy: Jung, Deleuze, Sexual Difference*

Jung, Deleuze, and the Problematic Whole

This book of expert essays explores the concept of the whole as it operates within the psychology of Jung, the philosophy of Deleuze, and selected areas of wider twentieth-century Western culture, which provided the context within which these two seminal thinkers worked.

Addressing this topic from a variety of perspectives and disciplines and with an eye to contemporary social, political, and environmental crises, the contributors aim to clarify some of the epistemological and ethical issues surrounding attempts, such as those of Jung and Deleuze, to think in terms of the whole, whether the whole in question is a particular bounded system (such as an organism, person, society, or ecosystem) or, most broadly, reality as a whole.

Jung, Deleuze, and the Problematic Whole will contribute to enhancing critical self-reflection among the many contemporary theorists and practitioners in whose work thinking in terms of the whole plays a significant role.

Roderick Main, PhD, is a professor in the Department of Psychosocial and Psychoanalytic Studies and Director of the Centre for Myth Studies at the University of Essex, UK.

Christian McMillan, PhD, is Lecturer at West Suffolk College, University of Suffolk, and was formerly Senior Research Officer in the Department for Psychosocial and Psychoanalytic Studies, University of Essex, UK.

David Henderson, PhD, is Lecturer in Jungian Studies in the Department for Psychosocial and Psychoanalytic Studies, University of Essex, UK. He is a member of the British Jungian Analytic Association (BJAA) and the International Association for Analytical Psychology (IAAP).

PHILOSOPHY & PSYCHOANALYSIS BOOK SERIES
JON MILLS
Series Editor

Philosophy & Psychoanalysis is dedicated to current developments and cutting-edge research in the philosophical sciences, phenomenology, hermeneutics, existentialism, logic, semiotics, cultural studies, social criticism, and the humanities that engage and enrich psychoanalytic thought through philosophical rigor. With the philosophical turn in psychoanalysis comes a new era of theoretical research that revisits past paradigms while invigorating new approaches to theoretical, historical, contemporary, and applied psychoanalysis. No subject or discipline is immune from psychoanalytic reflection within a philosophical context including psychology, sociology, anthropology, politics, the arts, religion, science, culture, physics, and the nature of morality. Philosophical approaches to psychoanalysis may stimulate new areas of knowledge that have conceptual and applied value beyond the consulting room reflective of greater society at large. In the spirit of pluralism, *Philosophy & Psychoanalysis* is open to any theoretical school in philosophy and psychoanalysis that offers novel, scholarly, and important insights in the way we come to understand our world.

Titles in this series:

Innovations in Psychoanalysis: Originality, Development, Progress
Edited by Aner Govrin and Jon Mills

Holism: Possibilities and Problems
Edited by Christian McMillan, Roderick Main, and David Henderson

**Romantic Metasubjectivity Through Schelling and Jung:
Rethinking the Romantic Subject**
Gord Barentsen

Jung, Deleuze, and the Problematic Whole

Edited by Roderick Main,
Christian McMillan, and
David Henderson

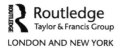
Routledge
Taylor & Francis Group

LONDON AND NEW YORK

First published 2021
by Routledge
2 Park Square, Milton Park, Abingdon, Oxon OX14 4RN

and by Routledge
52 Vanderbilt Avenue, New York, NY 10017

Routledge is an imprint of the Taylor & Francis Group, an informa business

British Library Cataloguing-in-Publication Data
A catalogue record for this book is available from the British Library

Library of Congress Cataloging-in-Publication Data
Names: Main, Roderick, editor. | Henderson, David, 1950– editor. |
McMillan, Christian, 1981– editor.
Title: Jung, Deleuze and the problematic whole / edited by
Roderick Main, Christian McMillan and David Henderson.
Description: Abingdon, Oxon : New York, NY : Routledge, 2020. |
Series: Philosophy and psychoanalysis |
Includes bibliographical references and index. |
Identifiers: LCCN 2020013446 (print) | LCCN 2020013447 (ebook) |
ISBN 9780367428747 (hardback) | ISBN 9780367428754 (paperback) |
ISBN 9780367855659 (ebook)
Subjects: LCSH: Whole and parts (Psychology) | Whole and parts (Philosophy) |
Holism. | Psychoanalysis and philosophy. | Jung, C. G. (Carl Gustav), 1875–1961. |
Deleuze, Gilles, 1925–1995.
Classification: LCC BF202 .J86 2020 (print) |
LCC BF202 (ebook) | DDC 150.19/54–dc23
LC record available at https://lccn.loc.gov/2020013446
LC ebook record available at https://lccn.loc.gov/2020013447

ISBN: 978-0-367-42874-7 (hbk)
ISBN: 978-0-367-42875-4 (pbk)
ISBN: 978-0-367-85565-9 (ebk)

Typeset in Times New Roman
by Newgen Publishing UK

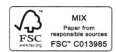

MIX
Paper from
responsible sources
FSC
www.fsc.org   FSC® C013985

Printed in the United Kingdom
by Henry Ling Limited

Contents

List of figures   ix
About the contributors   x
Acknowledgement   xiv

Introduction   1
RODERICK MAIN, CHRISTIAN McMILLAN, AND
DAVID HENDERSON

1   The ethical ambivalence of holism: An exploration
    through the thought of Carl Jung and Gilles Deleuze   20
    RODERICK MAIN

2   The 'image of thought' and the State-form in Jung's
    'The undiscovered self' and Deleuze and Guattari's
    'Treatise on nomadology'   51
    CHRISTIAN McMILLAN

3   Jung as symptomatologist   80
    DAVID HENDERSON

4   One, two, three... one: The edusemiotic self   102
    INNA SEMETSKY

5   The geometry of wholeness   125
    GEORGE HOGENSON

6   The status of exceptional experiences in the
    Pauli-Jung conjecture   142
    HARALD ATMANSPACHER

7   Holistic enchantment and eternal recurrence:
    Anaxagoras, Nietzsche, Deleuze, Klages, and Jung on
    the beauty of it all   167
    PAUL BISHOP

8   Holism and chance: Markets and meaning under
    neoliberalism   193
    JOSHUA RAMEY

    Index   209

Figures

4.1   Multiplicity   108
4.2   Tarot as a sign-system   121
5.1   Client's first sketch   126
5.2   Client's second sketch   127
5.3   Kalachakra mandala   128
5.4   Codex Fejérváry-Mayer   129
5.5   'The River Map', one of the legendary foundations
      of the *I Ching*   130
5.6   Mandala based on a woman's dream   131
5.7   The Mandelbrot set   134
5.8   Bifurcation graph   135
5.9   Bifurcation and Mandelbrot set   136
5.10 Cobweb plot   137
5.11 The initial stage   137
5.12 The final point of unity   138
5.13 Chaos   138
6.1   The mental, the physical, and the underlying,
      psychophysically neutral, holistic reality, according
      to the Pauli-Jung conjecture   145
6.2   Four fundamental classes of exceptional experiences
      resulting from the conceptual framework of the
      Pauli-Jung conjecture   156

About the contributors

Harald Atmanspacher, PhD, is a senior scientist and has been a staff member at Collegium Helveticum, University of Zurich and ETH Zurich, since 2007. After his PhD in physics at Munich University (1986), he worked as a research scientist at the Max Planck Institute for Extraterrestrial Physics at Garching until 1998. Then he served as head of the theory group at the Institute for Frontier Areas of Psychology at Freiburg until 2013. His fields of research are the theory of complex systems, conceptual and theoretical aspects of (algebraic) quantum theory, and mind–matter relations from inter-disciplinary perspectives. He is the president of the Society for Mind-Matter Research and editor-in-chief of the interdisciplinary international journal *Mind and Matter*.

Paul Bishop, PhD, is William Jacks Chair of Modern Languages at the University of Glasgow and his research has focused on the history of ideas in general and the German intellectual tradition in particular. His most recent publications include *On the Blissful Islands: With Nietzsche and Jung in the Shadow of the Superman* (Routledge, 2016) and, aside from his interests in translation and in the use of languages for business, he has published an introductory study on the thought of Klages entitled *Ludwig Klages and the Philosophy of Life: A Vitalist Toolkit* (Routledge, 2017).

David Henderson, PhD, is Lecturer in Jungian Studies at the Department for Psychosocial and Psychoanalytic Studies, University of Essex. He is a member of the British Jungian Analytic Association (BJAA) and the International Association for Analytical Psychology (IAAP). He is a convenor and regular contributor to the Jung-Lacan

Research Network. He has contributed chapters to *Re-Encountering Jung: Analytical Psychology and Contemporary Psychoanalysis* (Routledge, 2017; R.S. Brown, Ed.) and to *Depth Psychology and Mysticism*, (Palgrave, 2018; T. Cattoi and D. Orodisio, Eds.). Published papers include 'Freud and Jung: the creation of the psychoanalytic universe' and ' "A life free from care": the hermit and the analyst', both in *Psychodynamic Practice*. His book, *Apophatic Elements in the Theory and Practice of Psychoanalysis: Pseudo-Dionysius and C. G. Jung*, was published by Routledge in 2013. He was the co-investigator on a two-year (2016–18) research project titled ' "One world": logical and ethical implications of holism' funded by the Arts and Humanities Research Council, UK.

George Hogenson, PhD, teaches in the Analyst Training Program at the C.G. Jung Institute of Chicago and supervises trainees in the program. He regularly lectures on Jung's theories in the United States and Europe, and writes on the theory of archetypes, synchronicity, and the role of symbolism in the life of the individual. His work on the nature of archetypal imagery resulted in his being invited to present the Caroline and Earnest Fay Lectures at Texas A&M University in 2011. In addition to his work as a teacher and analyst, he is a former Vice President of the International Association for Analytical Psychology, and on the editorial board of *The Journal of Analytical Psychology*, to which he has contributed numerous articles.

Roderick Main, PhD, is a professor in the Department of Psychosocial and Psychoanalytic Studies and Director of the Centre for Myth Studies at the University of Essex. His publications include *The Rupture of Time: Synchronicity and Jung's Critique of Modern Western Culture* (Brunner-Routledge, 2004), *Revelations of Chance: Synchronicity as Spiritual Experience* (SUNY, 2007), *Jung on Synchronicity and the Paranormal* (Routledge/Princeton, 1997), and *Myth, Literature, and the Unconscious* (Karnac, 2013). He was principal investigator on a two-year (2016–18) research project titled ' "One world": logical and ethical implications of holism' funded by the Arts and Humanities Research Council, UK.

Christian McMillan, PhD was Senior Research Officer in the Department for Psychosocial and Psychoanalytic Studies at the University of Essex working on an AHRC-funded project ' "One world": logical and ethical implications of holism' (2016–18). His doctoral thesis, 'The image of thought in Jung's whole-Self: a critical study' (2014) focused on similarities and differences in the thought of depth psychologist C. G. Jung and French post-structuralist philosopher, Gilles Deleuze. Publications include: 'Jung, litera-ture, and aesthetics' in *Jung and Philosophy* (Routledge, 2019; Jon Mills, Ed.); 'Jung and Deleuze: enchanted openings to the other', *International Journal of Jungian Studies* (December 2018); 'Archetypal intuition: Beyond the human' in *Psychoanalysis, Culture and Society* (ed. David Henderson, 2012). Forthcoming publications include: 'Kant's influence on Jung's vitalism in the *Zofingia Lectures*' in *Holism: Possibilities and Problems* (C. McMillan, R. Main, and D. Henderson, Eds.; Routledge, 2020).

Joshua Ramey, PhD, is Visiting Assistant Professor of Peace, Justice, and Human Rights at Haverford College, USA. His work includes *The Hermetic Deleuze: Philosophy and Spiritual Ordeal* (Duke University Press, 2012) and *Politics of Divination: Neoliberal Endgame and the Religion of Contingency* (Rowman & Littlefield, 2016). He is co-editor, with Matthew Haar Farris, of *Speculation, Heresy, and Gnosis in Contemporary Philosophy of Religion: The Enigmatic Absolute* (Rowman & Littlefield, 2016).

Inna Semetsky has a PhD in educational philosophy preceded by an MA in counselling psychology and a GradDipEd. She has published eleven books including *Deleuze, Education and Becoming* (Sense, 2006), *Re-Symbolization of the Self* (Sense, 2011), *The Edusemiotics of Images* (Sense, 2013), and *Semiotic Subjectivity in Education and Counseling: Learning with the Unconscious* (Routledge, 2020). In 2000 she received the Kevelson Award from the Semiotic Society of America for her paper 'The adventures of a postmodern fool'. Her book *Edusemiotics* (Springer, 2015, co-authored) received the Book Award from the Philosophy of Education Society of Australasia. She has numerous book chapters including in the volume *Deleuze* *and the Schizoanalysis of Religion* (Bloomsbury, 2016; F. L. Shults and R. Powell-Jones, Eds.) as well as in international handbooks. Her papers have appeared in *Educational Philosophy and Theory*, *Zygon*, *Semiotica*, and other journals. She serves as a chief consultant to the recently established Institute for Edusemiotic Studies (Melbourne). She is also a long-time Tarot reader.

Acknowledgement

Work on this book was supported by the Arts and Humanities Research Council, UK [AH/N003853/1].

Introduction

Roderick Main, Christian McMillan,
and David Henderson

This book explores the concept of the whole as it operates within the
psychology of Carl Gustav Jung (1875–1961), the philosophy of Gilles
Deleuze (1925–1995), and selected areas of wider twentieth-century
Western culture, which provided the context within which Jung and
Deleuze worked. Addressing this topic from a variety of perspectives
and disciplines, the book aims to clarify some of the epistemological
and ethical issues surrounding attempts, such as those of Jung and
Deleuze, to think in terms of the whole, whether the whole in question
is a particular bounded system (such as an organism, person, society,
or ecosystem) or, most broadly, reality as a whole.

While reflection on the concept of the whole and its relations to
the elements that constitute the whole has been a staple of Western
philosophical and cultural traditions since the ancient Greeks (Dusek
1999: 19–22; Esfeld 2003: 10), such reflection has had, from the beginning of the twentieth century, several moments of particular salience.
The significance of wholeness was much discussed, for example, in the
life and mind sciences as well as in the physical sciences of the first
half of the twentieth century, especially within the German-speaking
world (Harrington 1996) but also more broadly (Lawrence and Weisz
1998). Ideas about wholeness were later a prominent influence on the
countercultural movements of the 1960s and 1970s (Wood 2010), and
continue to be so in the alternative spiritualities, therapies, and work
practices that have proliferated since the 1980s (Hanegraaff 1998;
Heelas and Woodhead 2005). Concern with how to think in terms of
wholes also underpins much of the current preoccupation with complexity theory (Cambray 2009), transdisciplinarity (Nicolescu 2002,

2008; Rowland 2017), and, certainly not least, ecology (Marietta 1994; Fellows 2019).

In most of these contexts, concern with the concept of the whole has been both epistemological and ethical. On the one hand, scientists and researchers have been taxed with how to acquire adequate knowledge and understanding of phenomena, such as those relating to life, consciousness, or culture, whose complexity does not readily lend itself to the kind of reductive analyses that have proven so successful in physics and chemistry (Phillips 1976). On the other hand, cultural commentators have argued that many of the environmental, political, economic, social, and psychological problems besetting the modern world have their deep roots in forms of thinking that embed divisive and fragmenting dualisms – for example, between humans and nature, spirit and matter, Creator and creation – and have advanced concepts of wholeness as means to foster a greater sense of interconnectedness, reconciliation, and unity (Berman 1981; Hanegraaff 1998: 119).

Perspectives giving central importance to the concept of the whole have also acquired, especially in the English-speaking world, an influential new moniker: holism (Smuts 1926). Coined by Jan Smuts in 1926, the term 'holism' and its adjectival form 'holistic' are now used, with varying emotional loading and varying degrees of clarity and emphasis, in practically every area of contemporary life, including academic as well as popular contexts (Main, McMillan, and Henderson 2020: 1–6). Reflecting this widespread usage, the terms 'holism' and 'holistic' are also used at many points in the present work, even though Jung seems never to have employed the German translation of holism (*Holismus*) nor Deleuze its French translation (*holisme*) – they wrote instead in terms of the German and French words for 'the whole': *die Ganzheit* (and its cognates) and *le Tout*, respectively.

Whether dubbed holism or not, thinking in terms of the whole has a presence in recent and contemporary academic and popular thought that could benefit from being more fully examined. Despite the salience their ideas have achieved in some quarters, advocates of holistic thinking have been charged with unrealisable epistemological ambitions, with misrepresenting reductionism, and with logical absurdity (Phillips 1976), as well as with claiming desirable outcomes, such as environmental outcomes, that are attributable to other factors (James 2007). Again, contrary to the claims that holistic thinking has beneficial ethical and political implications because of its reconciliation of deleterious dualisms, other commentators have charged holism with fostering 'totalitarian intuitions' (Popper 1957: 73). Again, the irony has not gone unnoticed that Smuts himself, for all that he promoted unity and wholeness on the highest international stage through his involvement in establishing both the League of Nations after the First World War and the United Nations after the Second World War, nevertheless was a proponent of segregation between whites and blacks in his home country of South Africa (Shelley 2008: 103). Although attempts have been made to address these epistemological and ethical criticisms (Bailis 1984–85; Harrington 1996), there continues to be deep intellectual suspicion of holistic perspectives.

With these and related issues in mind, the present book is a contribution towards clarifying the status of holistic thought through comparing relevant aspects of the work of Jung and Deleuze.[1] In focusing on Jung and Deleuze we have selected two influential twentieth-century thinkers whose work has in crucial respects been governed by the concept of the whole. For Jung, psychological wholeness, signified by the archetype of the self, was the goal of individual development, abetted where necessary by therapy (1928, 1944). Furthermore, in his later work he theorised that the wholeness whose realisation was aimed at was not just psychological but included also the world beyond the individual psyche: psyche and matter were considered two aspects of a single underlying reality which he referred to as the *unus mundus* or 'one world' (1955–56: §662). The process of realising wholeness was for Jung central not only to therapy and individual development but also to addressing many social, cultural, and political ills, which he considered largely to stem from thinking in a one-sidedly conscious (usually materialistic and rationalistic) way, without taking due account of the unconscious (1957). In his early work, the concept of the whole was an implicit concern for Jung, inasmuch as his work at that time was devoted to understanding what could be considered the opposite of wholeness, namely, psychic fragmentation that manifested as pathology (Smith 1990: 27–46). However, from the time of the experiences that led to his writing *The Red Book* (2009), wholeness became increasingly explicit as the central focus of Jung's psychological model and psychotherapy, and in the guise of the concepts of individuation and the self it pervades all of his mature writing.

Compared to Jung, Deleuze had a more conspicuously ambivalent relationship to the concept of the whole. On the one hand, he was relentlessly critical of organicistic thinking – often taken as synonymous with holism – in which the parts of a system are all considered to work towards the ends of the whole, like organs within an organism (Deleuze and Guattari 1972: 43). On the other hand, his entire opus was driven by the attempt to articulate a philosophy of pure immanence in which being was considered 'univocally', that is, not to be 'realer' in some expressions (e.g., as thinking, as consciousness, or as the Creator) than in others (e.g., as extension, as matter, or as creatures) (Deleuze 1968b, 2001). Within such a philosophy, reality could be conceptualised as an open and ever-changing whole in which the parts, even though not all internally related as in an organism, are, by dint of their involvement in a single 'plane of immanence', capable of being endlessly interrelated externally, horizontally, or, in the term Deleuze (and his co-writer Félix Guattari [1930–1992]) may have borrowed from Jung, 'rhizomatically' (Deleuze and Guattari 1991: 35–60; Somers-Hall 2012: 6–7). For Deleuze, such a conception of the open whole removed the need to conceive of an organising principle (e.g., mind, God) that is transcendent to what it organises (e.g., matter, the world). This had wide-ranging ethical and political implications for Deleuze, since he considered transcendence – the conception of a dimension of reality that was separate from and superior in being and value to the rest of reality – to be the root of totalitarian and other forms of exclusionary thought through providing a locus where privileged values and aspects of identity could order the rest of reality while themselves remaining shielded from criticism (1968a). The concept of the whole as such appears episodically in Deleuze's publications. It is explicit in *Bergsonism* (1966), the two cinema books (1983, 1985), the revision of *Proust and Signs* (1972), and in *Anti-Oedipus* (1972) and *What is Philosophy?* (1991), the latter two co-authored with Guattari. But expressed or at least implicated in other terms, such as 'the virtual', 'univocity of being', 'the plane of immanence', or the 'body without organs', the concept of the whole is arguably ubiquitous in Deleuze's writings.

Bringing together the work of Jung and Deleuze is by no means an easy or obvious task. In the first place, neither the ideas of Jung nor those of Deleuze can be easily or stably assimilated to established mainstream systems of thought that might provide secure reference points for comparison. Jung was avowedly not a systematic thinker (1939: ix), he acknowledged that he purposely wrote in an ambiguous style (1976: 70), and he regularly both drew on and expressed himself in the language of obscure esoteric currents of thought such as Gnosticism and alchemy (1929–54, 1944, 1946, 1951, 1955–56). Deleuze, for his part, when he drew on earlier philosophers, tended to give their ideas creative new interpretations, as in his treatment of Spinoza's concept of substance (1968b) or Nietzsche's doctrine of eternal recurrence (1962, 1968a). Even more challengingly, when he wrote in his own voice (or collaboratively with Guattari), he seemed often to overhaul his entire conceptual language from one publication to the next (Somers-Hall 2012: 1). In the second place, it is not obvious that the intellectual trajectories of the two thinkers should significantly intersect. Where Jung was a psychologist working in Switzerland in a predominantly German-speaking intellectual environment, Deleuze was a philosopher working in France in a predominantly Francophone milieu. Moreover, Jung was fifty years Deleuze's senior and thus of a different era, the pair never met, and the intellectual influence between them, such as it was, ran only one way, somewhat stealthily (Kerslake 2007: 70), from Jung to Deleuze.

However, the parallels and overlaps between Jung and Deleuze are nonetheless notable. Although a psychologist, Jung read deeply in philosophy, including thinkers and traditions that were also important to Deleuze, such as Kant, Nietzsche, and Western esotericism. Conversely, Deleuze, although a philosopher, explored deeply and commented critically on the concept of the unconscious and the field of psychoanalysis, including the work of Freud, Lacan, Klein, and Jung (Deleuze and Guattari 1972; Holland 2012). Both Jung and Deleuze worked in opposition to the mainstream in their respective disciplines, both were concerned with the relationship between personal transformation and knowledge ('gnosis'), and both were deeply critical of contemporary Western culture and politics.

Only a few prior works have explored the connections between Jung and Deleuze in any detail. Of seminal importance among these is Christian Kerslake's *Deleuze and the Unconscious* (2007), which meticulously uncovers the substantial influence of Jung on Deleuze's development of a conception of the unconscious that had more affinity with symbolist and occultist thought and the work of Janet and Bergson than with Freud's psychoanalysis. Although Deleuze was not explicit about this Jungian influence, Kerslake shows that it continued 'to shape his theory of the unconscious right up to *Difference and Repetition*' (ibid.: 69). Nor, arguably, is Kerslake's book important only for enriching understanding of Deleuze; it has also recently been hailed as '[t]he real turning point for a more comprehensive understanding of Jung's theorizing' (Hogenson 2019: 692).

Also significant, in this case for demonstrating the productivity of jointly applying the ideas of Jung and Deleuze, are works by Inna Semetsky and Barbara Jenkins. Semetsky, in a series of books going back over a decade, has applied concepts from Jung and Deleuze in developing a theory of 'edusemiotics', on the role of signs and their interpretation in education. Her focus has been sometimes on Deleuze (Semetsky 2006), sometimes on Jung (Semetsky 2013), and sometimes on both (Semetsky 2011, 2020). No less insightfully, Jenkins (2016) has drawn on both thinkers to offer a highly original exploration of how the 'social relations between things' can illuminate the role of desire and sexual difference in culture and the economy.

Kerslake's, Semetsky's, and Jenkins's books touch on many issues germane to the concept of the whole, but it is not their main focus. The same can be said of the various shorter discussions of connections between Jung and Deleuze that have been slowly increasing in number over the past couple of decades (e.g., Hauke 2000: 80–83; Kazarian 2010; Pint 2011; Holland 2012; Semetsky and Ramey 2013; Henderson 2014: 113–18; Cambray 2017; Hogenson 2019). There have also been several substantial works that have addressed the concept of the whole and/or holism either in Jung (Smith 1990; Kelly 1993; Huskinson 2004; Cambray 2009) or, albeit often via implicated terms rather than directly, in Deleuze (Ansell-Pearson 1999, 2007; Badiou 2000; Hallward 2006; Ramey 2012; Justaert 2012). However, these works have not brought the two thinkers together.

Most relevant to the present book are several works that were either a prelude to or part of the same overall project. The prelude was a study by McMillan (2015), which undertook a Deleuzian critique of Jung's concept of the whole and compellingly flagged some potential ethical problems with Jung's formulations, raising the question of whether and how these problems might be addressed. In a later work, focusing on late nineteenth- and early twentieth-century debates about vitalism that were of interest to both Jung and Deleuze, McMillan identified the importance of relations of interiority or exteriority in determining different kinds of holism and their ethical implications (McMillan 2020). The relations of interiority in organicistic holism imply that the whole is pre-given and closed, which could potentially give rise to forms of totalitarian and exclusionary thought. In Deleuze's criticisms of organicism and postulation of relations of exteriority, McMillan argues, it is possible to identify an alternative form of rhizomatic or 'transversal' holism, as well as a corresponding 'material vitalism', in which the whole remains always open and creative (ibid.: 122–23). Despite Jung's affinity with a range of premodern organicistic thinkers, his own dynamic concept of the whole can, McMillan argues (2018, 2019), also be understood as open and creative, with concepts such as psychic reality (*esse in anima*), the psychoid archetype, and synchronicity providing openings onto relations of exteriority. These studies show how an encounter between Jung's psychology and Deleuze's philosophy can foster an enhanced reflexivity in both, ensuring that any holism ascribed to these thinkers is a critical holism, one that challenges rather than reinforces the boundaries of systems.

In a paper complementary to his chapter in the present volume, Main (2017) has argued that, contrary to disenchantment, which is rooted in the metaphysics of theism whereby nature and the divine are considered ontologically separate, much holistic thought, including Jung's, has its roots in panentheistic metaphysics, in which nature is considered to be an expression or aspect of the divine. This metaphysics underpins, usually implicitly, many of the positive claims made for holism in relation to, for example, ecology, healthcare, education, social and political relations, and spirituality. It also, negatively for some, associates holism with heterodox traditions of Hermetic and mystical thought. In this context, both Main (2019) and McMillan (2018) have discussed the relevance for holism of Jung's concept of synchronicity – which is also a feature of several essays in the present volume (Semetsky, Hogenson, and Atmanspacher).

Also complementary to the present book is the same team of editors' *Holism: Possibilities and Problems* (McMillan, Main, and Henderson 2020). This companion volume focuses specifically on the concept of holism, and it encompasses a wider range of theoretical perspectives than just those of Jung and Deleuze, although the latter are well represented. The present book, however, is the first to focus specifically and in depth on the problem of the whole as it jointly figures in the works of Jung and Deleuze.

The contributors to the present book, as already noted, are all experts on the thought of either Jung or Deleuze, if not both. All are, or have been, academics, while some are also practitioners (Henderson, Hogenson, Semetsky, Ramey). Between them they represent a significant array of disciplines: philosophy (Ramey), psychotherapy/analysis (Henderson, Hogenson), education (Semetsky), physics (Atmanspacher), German studies (Bishop), and psychosocial and psychoanalytic studies (Main, McMillan). Some of the contributed essays explore the tensions between Jung's and Deleuze's different concepts of the whole and their respective ethical implications (Main, McMillan, Bishop). Others use the two authors primarily to amplify each other's thought (Henderson, Semetsky, Atmanspacher). Others again focus on contexts or topics equally informed by or equally relevant to both authors (Ramey, Hogenson). Among the epistemological, ethical, and methodological questions relating to the concept of the whole that are raised by the essays are the following:

- What is the relationship between a particular concept of ultimate wholeness and the multiplicities of experience?
- Can unitary reality be experienced directly?
- What is the status of symbolic knowledge of the whole?
- What are the ethical (including social, cultural, and political) implications of different concepts of the whole?
- Is there an intrinsic relationship between concepts of the whole and totalitarian thinking?
- Is it possible to avoid totalitarian dangers of holism by developing a form of critical holism based on the concept of an open whole?
- What is gained for the thought of Jung and Deleuze by staging an encounter between them?
- Can psychotherapeutic concepts such as Jung's be usefully appropriated by a philosophy such as Deleuze's, and can philosophical concepts such as Deleuze's be usefully appropriated by a psychology such as Jung's?

- How do the preoccupations of Jung and Deleuze in relation to the whole connect with other thinkers (such as Kant, Bergson, Klages, and Pauli) and other fields (such as complexity theory, physics, political economy, esotericism, and cultural history)?

Considering the magnitude of the questions being posed, the answers given to them are inevitably partial and provisional, and each essay refracts the questions through the author's own specific preoccupations and expertise. Nevertheless, there are many convergences among the essays. Important points that connect several of the contributions, even if they do not explicitly connect them all, include, far from exhaustively: that for both Jung and Deleuze wholeness is important because it helps to keep thought open to creativity and relationship; that wholes, or even the ultimate whole, can be creatively expressed through symbols (including symptoms, signs, and images); that these symbols are generated by estranging 'encounters', whether with art, exceptional experiences, or expressions of otherness or the unconscious more generally, each of which disturbs static patterns of thought; that knowledge of the whole can be direct (through immanent experience) as well as symbolic; that in either case knowledge of the whole is transformative, making ethical demands on the knower; that symbols of the whole are not just conscious constructions but are expressions of a natural process; that attempts to reify symbols of the whole result in one-sided or static representational thinking, and attempts to capture the practice of generating symbols are vulnerable to institutional control; and that many paths lead back from thinking about the whole to traditions of esoteric and mystical thought.

There are, of course, many aspects of thinking in terms of the whole that this book, largely for contingent reasons, has not been able to address as fully as we would have liked. The two most significant omissions are probably gender issues (useful resources would be Jenkins 2016 and Rowland 2017) and issues relating to environmentalism and the Anthropocene (see, for example, Fellows 2019). Another neglected topic is the relation between holistic thinking and Eastern thought (see, however, Yama 2020 and Main 2019: 67–68). Additional work could be usefully undertaken in each of these areas, as well as many others. Meanwhile, we hope that the following essays will, each in its way, spur further reflection both on the problem of the whole and on the thought of Jung and Deleuze, especially as the two thinkers creatively connect with each other.

In the opening chapter,[2] Roderick Main examines the disputed ethical status of holism through comparing aspects of the thought of Jung and Deleuze on the concept of wholeness. He first highlights relevant holistic features of Jung's psychological model, especially the concepts of the self and *unus mundus* (one world), and traces the cultural and social benefits that are claimed to flow from such a version of holism. He then confronts Jung's model with Deleuze's more constructivist way of thinking about wholes and totality in terms of difference, multiplicity, and pure immanence, which aims to ensure that his concept of the whole remains open. The Deleuzian perspective arguably exposes a number of questionable philosophical assumptions and ethical implications in Jung's holism – especially concerning the notions of original and restored wholes, organicism, and internal relations, with their implicit appeals to transcendence. In order to assess whether this Deleuzian critique is answerable, Main focuses attention on the understanding of transcendence and immanence within each thinker's model. Distinguishing between theism, pantheism, and panentheism, he proposes that the metaphysical logic of panentheism can provide a framework that is capable of reconciling the two thinkers' concepts of the whole. In light of this, Jung's position turns out to be an ally of the Deleuzian critique whose real target is the kind of strong transcendence characteristic of classical theism, which both thinkers eschew.

Focusing more explicitly on political issues, Christian McMillan (Chapter 2) also explores conceptual affinities between Jung's work and that of Deleuze together with his co-writer Guattari. McMillan draws extensively from one of Jung's final essays, 'The undiscovered self (present and future)' (1957), which was first published after the two world wars and in the immediate aftermath of the Red Scare in the United States. Jung's essay is noteworthy for its critique of the role of the State in modern times. It analyses the ways in which the State organises and orientates thought in a one-sided, ethically deleterious manner that excludes alternative forms of organisation. McMillan parallels this with Deleuze's critical focus on the organisation and distribution of relations within thought systems, of which the State is one variation. In the first half of the chapter, McMillan examines various concepts that Jung presents in his essay: positive concepts such as 'individual' and 'whole man' and negative concepts such as 'mass man', 'statistical man', and 'State'. In the second half of the chapter, McMillan relates Jung's analysis of the ways in which thought is orientated by the abstract idea of the modern State to Deleuze's critique of the image of thought, which formed a crucial part of his *Difference and Repetition* (1968a).

The uncanny internal resonance between Jung's psychological theory and Deleuze's philosophy receives further scrutiny from David Henderson (Chapter 3). Through a discussion of Deleuze's concepts of symptomatology, percept, and minor literature, from his *Essays Critical and Clinical* (1993), Henderson demonstrates the rich potential of Deleuzian thought for amplifying elements of Jung's psychology. According to Deleuze, 'Authors, if they are great, are more like doctors than patients. We mean that they are themselves astonishing diagnosticians or symptomatologists' (1969: 237). Jung can be read in this way as a symptomatologist, a 'clinician of civilization', who discovered the collective unconscious and prescribed a renewed relationship with wholeness as a remedy for the personal, cultural, and collective 'dis-eases' of modern life. The percept is a type of *vision* or *hearing*, and Henderson uses this concept of Deleuze's to reflect on Jung's capacity to *see* the unconscious. Finally, Henderson shows how Deleuze's concepts of minor literature and minority politics throw light on the corpus of Jung's writing and on the role of analytical psychology within the wider field of psychoanalysis.

Inna Semetsky (Chapter 4) continues the discussion of how symptoms, symbols, and signs can paradoxically express the unconscious or irrepresentable dimension of reality and thereby promote wholeness. She draws parallels between the axiom of the third-century alchemist Maria Prophetissa ('One becomes two, two becomes three, and out of the third comes the one as the fourth'), which Jung refers to as a metaphor for the process of individuation, and Deleuze's paradoxical logic of multiplicities (problematic Ideas) – both of which are based on the notion of the *tertium quid*, the included third. Semetsky argues that the reading of signs is an experiment that involves experiential learning (self-education or apprenticeship) and, ultimately, self-knowledge in the form of deep gnosis. Only through such knowledge can we become *in-dividual*, 'whole' selves. Semetsky's chapter also addresses ethics as the integration of the Jungian shadow archetype that may manifest in events of which, according to Deleuze, we must become worthy. To conclude, Semetsky presents an example of a transformative, healing ('making whole') practice that demonstrates the actualisation of the virtual archetypes via their 'dramatisation' in the esoteric yet 'real characters' of a neutral language, such as envisaged by Wolfgang Pauli, Jung's collaborator on the concept of synchronicity. By means of such a practice, for Semetsky, Deleuze's call to retrieve and read the structures immanent in the depth of the psyche is answered: we self-transcend by becoming-other.

Complementing Semetsky's appeal to esoteric thought, George Hogenson (Chapter 5) also explores the relationship between certain mathematical patterns and symbols of wholeness, but within a more scientific framework. He compares formally constructed mandalas and other geometric forms associated by Jung with the notion of wholeness with the iterative elaboration of the equations associated with Mandelbrot's fractal geometry. Hogenson argues that these symbols of wholeness are manifestations of fundamental mathematical structures that manifest throughout the natural world and connect psyche to the rest of nature in a fundamental form. Additionally, his analysis illustrates how the breakdown of psychic wholeness can be modelled in the breakdown of unity into chaotic states, thereby providing an argument for Jung's model of the psyche moving from the individual complex to the *unus mundus* and the unity of the self.

In an argument also thoroughly grounded in science, in this case physics and consciousness research, Harald Atmanspacher (Chapter 6) explores relational and immanent experiences in relation to what he has called the Pauli-Jung conjecture, which is a coherent reconstruction of Pauli's and Jung's scattered ideas about the relationship between the mental and the physical and their common origin. It belongs to the decompositional variety of dual-aspect monisms, in which a basic, psychophysically neutral reality is conceived of as radically holistic, without distinctions, and hence discursively inexpressible. Epistemic domains such as the mental and the physical emerge from this base reality by differentiation. Within this conceptual framework, Atmanspacher identifies three different options to address so-called exceptional experiences, that is, deviations from typical reality models that individuals develop and utilise to cope with their environment.

Such experiences can be understood (i) as either mental images or physical events, (ii) as relations between the mental and the physical, and (iii) as direct experiences of the psychophysically neutral reality. These three classes are referred to as reified, relational, and immanent experiences.

Paul Bishop (Chapter 7) is also concerned with ideas and experiences that express a holistic and enchanted view of reality. He argues that for Friedrich Nietzsche – a key influence on Jung and Deleuze alike – the world is both disenchanted and enchanted. From a transcendental perspective (associated with Judeo-Christianity), the world is disenchanted; it is 'the work of a suffering and tormented God'. Yet from an immanent perspective, the world is in fact enchanted – or potentially so, and the means by which Nietzsche proposes to re-enchant (or rediscover the primordial enchantment of) the world is the doctrine of eternal recurrence. In *Thus Spoke Zarathustra*, his animals proclaim Zarathustra to be 'the teacher of the eternal recurrence', and this passage has caught the attention of numerous commentators, including Heidegger and Deleuze. Another critic of Nietzsche's doctrine of eternal recurrence is Ludwig Klages, himself deeply invested in the challenges of disenchantment and re-enchantment. Central to Klages's philosophy are his doctrine of the 'reality of images' and his related notion of 'elementary similarity'. Elementary similarity informs the kind of perception he associates with *die Seele*, that is, with the soul or the psyche, and which he regards as essentially *symbolic*. Can the concepts of identity, similarity, dissimilarity, and difference, Bishop asks, help us to relate and coordinate the thought of Klages, Jung, and Deleuze – and not just in relation to Nietzsche?

The volume concludes with Joshua Ramey's highly original perspective on the relationship between divination and financial markets (Chapter 8). Ramey explores how extreme variants of neoliberal ideology about the power of markets, particularly as articulated in the late work of Friedrich Hayek, produce illusions about the kind of meanings that can be construed on the basis of chance or random processes. Randomness poses an interesting problem for holism in general, but here Ramey focuses on the specific power that uncertainty (linked to the basic fact of extreme contingency, or chance) is supposed to display, within 'correctly' functioning markets, to generate meaning. In Ramey's book, *Politics of Divination: Neoliberal Endgame and the*

Religion of Contingency (2016), he has argued that the extreme version of neoliberal market apologetics holds that markets can function as divination processes – that is, as inquiries into more-than-human knowledge. The complex and unstable relation between chance and the Whole is figured here in an equivocation over whether chance means everything or nothing, and helps to explain the particular relation between neoliberal ideology and nihilism.

Notes

1 The present volume is one of the outputs of a research project examining the logical and ethical implications of holism through comparing relevant aspects of the work of Jung and Deleuze. The project, run by the present editors, was titled ' "One world": logical and ethical implications of holism' and was funded by the Arts and Humanities Research Council, UK, between 2016 and 2018 (grant number AH/N003853/1). In brief, we wished to understand better why holism attracts such strong positive and negative valuations, and whether the positive or the negative point of view, if either, is the better warranted. We attempted to probe the underpinning concepts of ultimate wholeness at work in different models, such as those of Jung and Deleuze, and to trace how those concepts of wholeness might relate, ethically and politically as well as epistemologically, to the multiplicities of experience. We were especially concerned with the significance and impact of these issues in the field of psychotherapy. As part of the project, an invited group of experts in the thought of Jung and/or Deleuze presented and discussed papers in an intensive two-day workshop at the University of Essex, and it is those papers which in revised form are the basis of this book. One of the participants at the workshop, Christian Kerslake, was unfortunately unable to contribute an essay, but the volume has nevertheless greatly benefited from his comments during the workshop, as well as from the inspiration provided by his ground-breaking book, *Deleuze and the Unconscious* (2007). The workshop was followed by an international conference, also at the University of Essex, with a broader remit on holism more generally and much wider participation. Some of the papers from that conference, as well as our more general findings about holism, have been published in a companion volume to the present book (McMillan, Main, and Henderson 2020; Main, McMillan, and Henderson 2020).
2 The following summary of the chapters is based on abstracts provided by the contributors.

References

(In the citations and reference list, dates within parentheses refer to the date of original publication. The date of edition consulted, if different, appears after the publisher in the reference list.)

Ansell-Pearson, K. (1999). *Germinal Life: The Difference and Repetition of Deleuze*. London and New York: Routledge.

Ansell-Pearson, K. (2007). Beyond the human condition: An introduction to Deleuze's lecture course. *SubStance #114 36*(3): 57–71.

Badiou, A. (2000). *Deleuze: The Clamor of Being* (L. Churchill, Trans.). Minneapolis, MN: University of Minnesota Press.

Bailis, S. (1984–85). Against and for holism: A reply and a rejoinder to D. C. Phillips. *Issues in Integrative Studies 3*: 17–41.

Berman, M. (1981). *The Reenchantment of the World*. Ithaca, NY: Cornell University Press.

Cambray, J. (2009). *Synchronicity: Nature and Psyche in an Interconnected Universe*. College Station, TX: Texas A and M University Press.

Cambray, J. (2017). The emergence of the ecological mind in Hua-Yen/Kegon Buddhism and Jungian psychology. *Journal of Analytical Psychology 62*(1): 20–31.

Deleuze, G. (1962). *Nietzsche and Philosophy* (H. Tomlinson, Trans.). London: Bloomsbury, 2006.

Deleuze, G. (1966). *Bergsonism* (H. Tomlinson and B. Habberjam, Trans.). New York: Zone Books, 1991.

Deleuze, G. (1968a). *Difference and Repetition* (P. Patton, Trans.). London: Bloomsbury, 2014.

Deleuze, G. (1968b). *Expressionism in Philosophy: Spinoza* (M. Joughin, Trans.). New York: Zone, 2013.

Deleuze, G. (1969). *The Logic of Sense* (C. Boundas, Ed.; M. Lester and C. Stivale, Trans.). New York: Columbia University Press, 1990.

Deleuze, G. (1972). *Proust and Signs: The Complete Text* (R. Howard, Trans.). London: Athlone, 2000; original French publication 1964).

Deleuze, G. (1983). *Cinema 1: The Movement-Image* (H. Tomlinson and B. Habberjam, Trans.). London: Athlone Press, 1992.

Deleuze, G. (1985). *Cinema 2: The Time-Image* (H. Tomlinson and R. Galeta, Trans.). Minneapolis: University of Minnesota Press, 1989.

Deleuze, G. (1993). *Essays Critical and Clinical* (D. Smith and M. Greco, Trans.). Minneapolis: University of Minnesota Press, 1998.

Deleuze, G. (2001). *Pure Immanence: Essays on a Life*. New York: Zone.

Deleuze, G., and Guattari, F. (1972). *Anti-Oedipus: Capitalism and Schizophrenia* (R. Hurley, M. Seem, and H. Lane, Trans.). Minneapolis: University of Minnesota Press, 2000.

Deleuze, G., and Guattari, F. (1991). *What is Philosophy?* (H. Tomlinson and G. Burchell, Trans.). New York: Columbia University Press, 1994.Dusek, V. (1999). *The Holistic Inspirations of Physics: The Underground History of Electromagnetic Theory.* New Brunswick, NJ: Rutgers University Press.

Esfeld, M. (2003). Philosophical holism. In *Encyclopedia of Life Support Systems.* Paris: UNESCO/Eolss Publishers [www.eolss.net].

Fellows, A. (2019). *Gaia, Psyche and Deep Ecology: Navigating Climate Change in the Anthropocene.* London and New York: Routledge.

Hallward, P. (2006). *Out of This World: Deleuze and the Philosophy of Creation.* London and New York: Verso.

Hanegraaff, W. (1998). *New Age Religion and Western Culture: Esotericism in the Mirror of Secular Thought.* Albany, NY: State University of New York Press.

Harrington, A. (1996). *Reenchanted Science: Holism in German Culture from Wilhelm II to Hitler.* Princeton, NJ: Princeton University Press.

Hauke, C. (2000). *Jung and the Postmodern: The Interpretation of Realities.* London and Philadelphia.

Heelas, P. and Woodhead, L., with B. Seel, B. Szeszynski, and K. Tusting (2005). *The Spiritual Revolution: Why Religion in Giving Way to Spirituality.* Oxford: Blackwell.

Henderson, D. (2014). *Apophatic Elements in the Theory and Practice of Psychoanalysis: Pseudo-Dionysius and C. G. Jung.* London and New York: Routledge.

Hogenson, G. (2019). The controversy around the concept of archetypes. *Journal of Analytical Psychology 64*(5): 682–700.

Holland, E. (2012). Deleuze and psychoanalysis. In D. Smith and H. Somers-Hall (Eds.), *The Cambridge Companion to Deleuze*, 307–36. Cambridge: Cambridge University Press.

Huskinson, L. (2004). *Nietzsche and Jung: The Whole Self in the Union of Opposites.* Hove and New York: Brunner-Routledge, 2004.

James, S. (2007). Against holism: Rethinking Buddhist environmental ethics. *Environmental Values 16*: 447–61.

Jenkins, B. (2016). *Eros and Economy: Jung, Deleuze, Sexual Difference.* London and New York: Routledge.

Jung, C. G. (1928). The relations between the ego and the unconscious. In *The Collected Works of C. G. Jung* (Sir H. Read, M. Fordham, and G. Adler, Eds.; W. McGuire, Exec. Ed.; R. F. C. Hull, Trans.) [hereafter *Collected*

Works], vol. 7, *Two Essays on Analytical Psychology*, 2nd ed., 121–241. London: Routledge and Kegan Paul, 1966.

Jung, C. G. (1929–54). *Collected Works,* vol. 13, *Alchemical Studies.* London: Routledge and Kegan Paul, 1968.

Jung, C. G. (1939). Foreword. In J. Jacobi, *The Psychology of C. G. Jung*, ix. London: Routledge and Kegan Paul, 1975.

Jung, C. G. (1944). *Collected Works,* vol. 12, *Psychology and Alchemy*, 2nd ed. London: Routledge and Kegan Paul, 1968.

Jung, C. G. (1946). The psychology of the transference. In *Collected Works,* vol. 16, *The Practice of Psychotherapy*, 2nd ed., 163–323. London: Routledge and Kegan Paul, 1966.

Jung, C. G. (1951). *Collected Works,* vol. 9ii, *Aion*, 2nd ed. London: Routledge and Kegan Paul, 1968.

Jung, C. G. (1955–56). *Collected Works,* vol. 14, *Mysterium Coniunctionis: An Inquiry into the Separation and Synthesis of Psychic Opposites in Alchemy*, 2nd ed. London: Routledge and Kegan Paul, 1970.

Jung, C. G. (1957). The undiscovered self (Present and future). In *Collected Works,* vol. 10, *Civilization in Transition*, 2nd ed., 245–305. London: Routledge and Kegan Paul, 1970.

Jung, C. G. (1976). *Letters 2: 1951–1961* (G. Adler and A. Jaffé, Eds.; R. F. C. Hull, Trans.). London: Routledge and Kegan Paul.

Jung, C. G. (2009). *The Red Book: Liber Novus* (S. Shamdasani, Ed.; M. Kyburz, J. Peck, and S. Shamdasani, Trans.). New York: W. W. Norton.

Justaert, K. (2012). *Theology After Deleuze*. London: Continuum.

Kazarian, E. (2010). The revolutionary unconscious: Deleuze and Masoch. *SubStance 39*(2): 91–106.

Kelly, S. (1993). *Individuation and the Absolute: Hegel, Jung and the Path Toward Wholeness*. New York: Paulist Press.

Kerslake, C. (2007). *Deleuze and the Unconscious*. London: Continuum.

Lawrence, C., and Weiss, G. (Eds.) (1998). *Greater than the Parts: Holism in Biomedicine 1920–1950*. Oxford: Oxford University Press.

Main, R. (2017). Panentheism and the undoing of disenchantment. *Zygon: Journal of Religion and Science 52*(4): 1098–122.

Main, R. (2019). Synchronicity and holism. In *Analytical Psychology Meets Academic Research: Avignon Conference 2018*, 59–74. *Revue de Psychologie Analytique* (Hors série).

Main, R., McMillan, C., and Henderson, D. (2020). Introduction. In C. McMillan, R. Main, and D. Henderson (Eds.), *Holism: Possibilities and Problems*, 1–14. London and New York: Routledge.

Marietta, D. (1994). *For People and the Planet: Holism and Humanism in Environmental Ethics*. Philadelphia, PA: Temple University Press.

McMillan, C. (2015). The 'image of thought' in Jung's 'Whole-Self': A critique. Unpublished PhD thesis, University of Essex, UK.

McMillan, C. (2018). Jung and Deleuze: Enchanted openings to the Other: A philosophical contribution. *International Journal of Jungian Studies 10*(3): 184–98.

McMillan, C. (2019). Jung, literature, and aesthetics. In J. Mills (Ed.), *Jung and Philosophy*, 269–88. London and New York: Routledge.

McMillan, C. (2020). Kant's influence on Jung's vitalism in the *Zofingia Lectures*. In C. McMillan, R. Main, and D. Henderson (Eds.), *Holism: Possibilities and Problems*, 118–29. London and New York: Routledge.

McMillan, C., Main, R., and Henderson, D. (Eds.) (2020). *Holism: Possibilities and Problems*. London and New York: Routledge.

Nicolescu, B. (2002). *Manifesto of Transdisciplinarity*. Albany, NY: State University of New York Press.

Nicolescu, B. (Ed.) (2008). *Transdisciplinarity: Theory and Practice*. Creskill, NJ: Hampton Press.

Phillips, D. C. (1976). *Holistic Thought in Social Science*. Stanford, CA: Stanford University Press.

Pint, K. (2011). Doubling back: Psychoanalytical literary theory and the perverse return to Jungian space. *S: Journal of the Jan van Eyck Circle for Lacanian Ideology Critique 4*: 47–55.

Popper, K. (1957). *The Poverty of Historicism*. London: Routledge.

Ramey, J. (2012). *The Hermetic Deleuze: Philosophy and Spiritual Ordeal*. Durham, NC: Duke University Press.

Ramey, J. (2016). *Politics of Divination: Neoliberal Endgame and the Religion of Contingency*. London and New York: Rowman and Littlefield.

Rowland, S. (2017). *Remembering Dionysus: Revisioning psychology and literature in C. G. Jung and James Hillman*. London and New York: Routledge.

Semetsky, I. (2006). *Deleuze, Education and Becoming*. Rotterdam, NL: Sense Publishers.

Semetsky, I. (2011). *Re-Symbolization of the Self: Human Development and Tarot Hermeneutic*. Rotterdam, NL: Sense Publishers.

Semetsky, I. (2013) (Ed.). *Jung and Educational Theory*. Oxford: Wiley-Blackwell.

Semetsky, I. (2020). *Semiotic Subjectivity in Education and Counseling: Learning with the Unconscious*. London and New York: Routledge.

Semetsky, I., and Ramey, J. (2013). Deleuze's philosophy and Jung's psychology: Learning and the unconscious. In I. Semetsky (Ed.), *Jung and Educational Theory*, 63–75. Oxford: Wiley-Blackwell.

Shelley, C. (2008). Jan Smuts and personality theory: The problem of holism in psychology. In R. Diriwächter and J. Valsiner (Eds.), *Striving for the*

Whole: Creating Theoretical Syntheses, 89–109. New Brunswick and London: Transaction Publishers.

Smith, C. (1990). *Jung's Quest for Wholeness: A Religious and Historical Perspective*. Albany, NY: State University of New York Press.

Smuts, J. C. (1926). *Holism and Evolution*. London: Macmillan.

Somers-Hall, H. (2012). Introduction. In D. Smith and H. Somers-Hall (Eds.), *The Cambridge Companion to Deleuze*, 1–12. Cambridge: Cambridge University Press.

Wood, L. S. (2010). *A More Perfect Union: Holistic Worldviews and the Transformation of American Culture after World War II*. Oxford: Oxford University Press.

Yama, M. (2020). The concept of *kami* in Shintō and holism: Psychotherapy and Japanese literature. In C. McMillan, R. Main, and D. Henderson (Eds.), *Holism: Possibilities and Problems*, 170–79. London and New York: Routledge.

Chapter 1

The ethical ambivalence of holism

An exploration through the thought of Carl Jung and Gilles Deleuze

Roderick Main

Among the many ways in which the concept of holism has been used since it was coined almost a hundred years ago (Smuts 1926), two polarised extremes stand out. On the one hand, holism – briefly, the doctrine that the whole is more than the sum of its parts[1] – has been championed as the solution to a range of scientific and cultural problems associated with the condition Max Weber termed disenchantment (1919: 139, 155). For example, as Anne Harrington has related, various life and mind scientists in the German-speaking world during the first decades of the twentieth century sought to develop 'a new science of Wholeness' that, as well as solving scientific problems that seemed intractable to an analytic approach, would counteract the cultural sense of alienation and meaninglessness that was seen as stemming from 'the old science of the Machine' with its 'mechanistic, instrumentalist thinking' (1996: xv–xvi). Later in the twentieth century, Morris Berman, lamenting how a disenchanted worldview had 'destroyed the continuity of the human experience and the integrity of the human psyche' and 'very nearly wrecked the planet as well', proposed holism as a key component in an urgently needed 're-enchantment of the world': '*Some* type of holistic, or participating, consciousness and a corresponding socio-political formation', he wrote, 'have to emerge if we are to survive as a species' (1981: 23). Similar sentiments also inform many of the more recent manifestations of holistic thought in spirituality, therapy, ecology, and other areas (Hanegraaff 1998: 119–58; Heelas and Woodhead 2005; Fellows 2019).

On the other hand, holism has been charged with facilitating the emergence of totalitarianism and its associated ills. Organicistic and other holistic tropes were part of the Nazi rhetoric, for instance, and for at least some scientists in the interwar German-speaking world there were very real connections between the holism promoted in their scientific work and their support for aspects of Nazi ideology, such as the expectation that individuals should subordinate their self-interest in order to serve the organic whole, the Volk, of which they were parts (Harrington 1996: 175–78). While Harrington notes that 'the history of German holism is a history of many stories and [...] other political relationships [than conservative, antidemocratic, and totalitarian ones] were possible, and in various ways, persuasive' (ibid.: 208), other commentators have argued that the connection between holism and totalitarianism is intrinsic. Karl Popper, for example, identified holism as one of the presuppositions, along with historicism and essentialism, that typically leads to totalitarian political formations (1945, 1957). More recently, Jozet Keulartz concluded a discussion of holism in the thought of Jan Christiaan Smuts, Alfred North Whitehead, and late twentieth-century ecology with the claim that 'the link between holism and totalitarianism does not rest exclusively on historical coincidence but may well be the consequence of an internal relationship' (1998: 141; see also Cooper 1996).

The ethical ambivalence that seems to attach to holism – where it is seen alternatively as the solution to a range of social, cultural, and political ills or as a major cause of such ills – is explored in the present chapter through an examination of the work of the Swiss psychologist Carl Gustav Jung (1875–1961). Jung's professional life overlapped with the emergence of the principal forms of both twentieth-century holism and twentieth-century totalitarianism. His work is itself deeply holistic (Smith 1990; Main 2019) and has been construed as, on the one hand, re-enchanting (Main 2011, 2013, 2017) and, on the other hand, problematically implicated with Nazism and anti-Semitism (Grossman 1979; Maidenbaum and Martin 1992). It thus exemplifies the problem under discussion.

The question that this chapter addresses, then, is what are the ethical implications of holism, and more particularly whether the case of Jung suggests that there is indeed an intrinsic relationship between holistic and totalitarian forms of thought. The approach taken to exploring these issues involves first highlighting salient aspects of Jung's holistic thought and the ethical benefits, individual and social, that arguably stem from it. This positive picture is then confronted with a perspective deeply critical of holistic thought and its possible totalitarian implications – the perspective of the French post-structuralist philosopher Gilles Deleuze (1925–1995).[2] Deleuze was demonstrably influenced by Jung and developed ideas that have many affinities with Jung's (Kerslake 2007; Holland 2012: 310–13), and he also, like Jung, reflected deeply on the problem of the whole throughout his professional life (Ansell-Pearson 2007: 5). This makes it all the more interesting that on the particular issue of holistic thought, Deleuze appears to have taken a position almost opposite to Jung's. Rather than pore over historical or biographical issues, however, the chapter examines some of the metaphysical assumptions underpinning Jung's and Deleuze's thought, particularly in relation to transcendence and immanence, in order to assess the extent to which Deleuze's criticisms of holistic thought as intrinsically totalitarian might be answerable from the perspective of Jung's holism. It also considers whether this confrontation has any implications for understanding the thought of Deleuze.

Jung's holistic thought

The appropriateness of designating Jung's work as a form of holism, despite his not having used this specific term himself,[3] is supported by a number of considerations that have been discussed elsewhere (Main 2019). These include the pivotal and pervasive importance of the concept of wholeness in his work; the parallels between his thought and that of contemporaneous thinkers widely designated as holists; his explicit influence on subsequent self-proclaimed holists; and the close fit of his ideas with various characterisations and formal definitions of holism (ibid.: 61–63). For the purpose of the present discussion, there are several points to highlight.

As a psychiatrist and psychotherapist, Jung's primary concern was with processes of psychological healing and development. Increased 'human wholeness' (1944: §32) was important to him because he envisaged this as the goal of those processes. He characterised such wholeness as consisting in a union of opposites (1911–12/1952: §460; 1946: §532; 1958: §784), most generally as 'the union of the conscious and unconscious personality' (1940: §294), and he designated this united state with the concept of the self (1955–56: §145), the 'archetype of wholeness' (1951a: §351; 1952a: §757). The self, or wholeness, found expression in a multitude of symbols for Jung, among which the mandala was of particular importance (1944: §§323–31). The overall process of developing such wholeness he called 'individuation' (1928: §§266–406). Jung's thought is holistic, then, in that it presupposes the possibility of psychological wholeness, and that presupposition informs both how psychological processes are understood and how psychotherapy is done.

While Jung was primarily concerned with psychological wholeness, he considered that the process of developing psychological wholeness could lead in the direction of a wider wholeness that included the world beyond the psyche. At one level, the world beyond the psyche included the social world. Jung was not a social holist in the usual sense of holding that social entities have properties that are irreducible to the behaviours of the individuals composing those social entities (1957: §§504, 553–54). Nevertheless, he considered that the pursuit of wholeness at the individual level, insofar as it 'makes us aware of the unconscious, which unites and is common to all mankind', could '[bring] to birth a consciousness of human community' (1945: §227). As he wrote in connection to this, 'Individuation [the process of realising the wholeness of the self] is an at-one-ment with oneself and at the same time with humanity, since oneself is a part of humanity' (ibid.).

At another level – or other levels – the world beyond the psyche included for Jung the physical and spiritual worlds. In the concluding chapter of his late work *Mysterium Coniunctionis* (1955–56: §§654–789), Jung presented his model of psychological development in terms of three 'conjunctions' (or a conjunction in three stages) as described by the sixteenth-century alchemist Gerhard Dorn. The first conjunction or stage was the union of the psyche and spirit, or of the mind within itself, a realisation of inner psychic integration (ibid.: §§669–76). The second conjunction or stage was the union of the integrated psyche with the body or with the world of physical reality (ibid.: §§677–93). The third and final conjunction or stage was the union of the integrated mind and body with the world of potential, the unitary source of all actualisations, the 'one world' or *unus mundus* (ibid.: §§759–75). This conception implied that realisation of wholeness could involve two forms of integration that were empirical or immanent: the integration of the mind within itself and the integration of the internally integrated mind with the body and with the external world. Besides this, however, the conception also implied that realisation of wholeness could involve a third form of integration that was non-empirical or transcendent: the integration of the integrated mind-body with its unitary source. At its deepest levels, Jung's holism was thus cosmic and mystical as well as psychological and social.

The possibility of holistic relations existing between, as well as at, different levels of reality is reflected in Jung sometimes suggesting that the relationship between psychological wholeness and the wholeness of humanity or of the world could be understood as one between microcosm and macrocosm. Jung sometimes invoked this idea in his discussions of society, describing the individual person as 'a social microcosm, reflecting on the smallest scale the qualities of society at large' (1957: §553; see also §540). More often, however, he introduced the idea in relation to the cosmological visions and transformative practices of pre-modern, non-Western, and especially esoteric, above all alchemical, thinkers (1944: §472; 1952b: §§923, 925–26, 928–29, 937).

Although Jung did not generally present his thinking about wholeness in terms of the relationship between wholes and parts, as do most formal definitions of holism (Phillips 1976: 6; Esfeld 2003), such terms and ways of understanding are arguably implicit in his view (Main 2019: 61–63). Like more explicitly holistic thinkers, Jung prioritised the perspective of wholeness when dealing with subject matter, in his case the human personality or more specifically the self, that could not be adequately understood in terms of a purely analytic approach (Jung 1952b: §§821, 864; Phillips 1976: 6–12). Like explicit holists, he saw this whole as more than the sum of its parts (Phillips 1976: 12–15); that is, the self was for him more than an aggregate of the contents comprising it: in shorthand, the conscious ego, the shadow, and the other archetypes of the collective unconscious (Jung 1944: §44; 1951a: §43; 1955–56: §145). He also considered that the self, as the whole, determined the nature of its parts (Phillips 1976: 16); that is, to the extent that it was the 'organiser of the personality' (Jung 1958: §694) the self determined the nature of the conscious ego, shadow, and other archetypes. Again like explicit holists, Jung did not think the parts could be understood if considered in isolation from the whole (Phillips 1976: 17–19);

in his terms, since the manifestations of the ego, shadow, and other archetypes at any time were related to their role in the process of individuation, which in turn was governed by the self (Jung 1928, 1944), it was not possible adequately to understand the ego, shadow, and other archetypes in isolation from the self. Finally, Jung saw the parts as dynamically interrelated or interdependent (Phillips 1976: 19); the ego, shadow, and other archetypes evinced for him precisely such interrelationship and interdependence, as described throughout his mature discussions of his psychology (1928; 1940: §302; 1944; 1955–56; see also Smith 1990; Cambray 2009: 33–36).

In sum, Jung's conception of wholeness, while primarily psychological, extended to include the social world, the physical world, and the spiritual world, and the connections among these various domains of experience were sometimes framed in terms of the relationship between microcosm and macrocosm. Although he did not use the term 'holism' himself, his concept of wholeness can be quite closely fitted with formal analytic definitions of holism.

The ethical implications of Jung's holistic thought

For Jung, attending to wholeness could generate not only certain kinds of knowledge but also distinct ethical benefits. At the individual level, the principal ethical benefit of attending to wholeness was that it enabled persons to address their one-sidedness and the pathologies that Jung considered to stem from one-sidedness (1937: §255, 258). By becoming more conscious of aspects of their whole personality that had been operating unconsciously, they would be less likely to project these aspects onto others (1951a: §16).

At the social level, we have already seen that Jung considered development towards wholeness of the self as a process that made individuals conscious of their shared collectivity (1945: §227). In a more specifically political register, he also argued that, insofar as the self or wholeness with which individuation brings a person into relationship transcends empirical experience (1957: §509; 1958: §779), it could serve, as belief in God had traditionally done, as an 'extramundane principle capable of relativising the overpowering influence of external [social and political] factors' and in particular could prevent a person's 'otherwise inevitable submersion in the mass' (1957: §511; see also

McMillan 2021). More widely still, in the light of his late concepts of synchronicity, the psychoid archetype, and the *unus mundus*, Jung suggested that there might be a universal interconnectedness among all aspects of reality, including between psyche and matter (both organic and inorganic) (1955–56: §§662, 767). This would have implications for human responsibility towards the natural as well as cultural and social environments (Fellows 2019).

Finally and most pertinently for the present discussion, Jung's holistic thought represented a response to the condition of disenchantment. For the wholeness promoted by Jung's psychological model involves the integration, or at least reconciliation or harmonising, of factors normally treated as separate and irreconcilable within the framework of disenchantment: irrationality and rationality, transcendence and immanence, value and fact, religion and science. Weber's fragmentary but influential statements about disenchantment imply, at least in an 'ideal-typical' case (Asprem 2014: 39–40), four main propositions. As concisely summarised by Egil Asprem, these are that there is no genuine mystery or magic, so that 'nature can in principle be understood by empiricism and reason [alone]' (2014: 36; Weber 1919: 139); that 'science can know nothing beyond the empirically given' and therefore 'metaphysics is impossible' (Asprem 2014: 36; Weber 1919: 140–42); that values cannot be derived from facts and hence 'science can know nothing of meaning' (Asprem 2014: 36; Weber 1919: 142–44, 146); and finally, because empiricism and reason provide no evidence for the putative transcendent realities and values of religion, that science and religion are irreconcilable and consequently one can only embrace religion by putting aside science, that is, by making an 'intellectual sacrifice' (Weber 1919: 155; Asprem 2014: 36).

Against this, Jung, with the inclusion in his holistic psychological model of the unconscious, the non-rational, and the irrepresentable, implied the impossibility of ever fully or adequately grasping nature by empiricism and reason alone (1963: 390; Main 2017: 1111). With his openness to anomalous, mystical, and other forms of numinous experiences, his understanding of symbols and myths as 'the revelation of a divine life in man' (1963: 373), and his formulation of transcendental concepts such as the archetype in itself, synchronicity, and the *unus mundus*, he implied (even while he may have denied) the possibility of metaphysics (Jung 1947/1954; 1952b; 1955–56: §§759–75; Main

2017: 1111–13). And with his inclusion, in order to achieve a 'whole judgement' (1952b: §961), of the functions of feeling and intuition and of a form of acausal connection through meaning (synchronicity), he implied the possibility of meaning and value, no less than of order and fact, being objective features of reality (Jung 1921, 1952b; Main 2017: 1113–14). Taken together these aspects further implied that religion and science were reconcilable and both contributed perspectives essential to a whole picture of the world (Main 2017: 1114–15). In thus comprehensively challenging disenchantment, Jung's holistic thought also challenged the ethical implications of disenchantment that so troubled many cultural commentators throughout the twentieth century (ibid.: 1001–2).

Deleuze's criticisms of holistic thought

Jung's crediting of anomalous and numinous experience, his willingness to develop concepts such as synchronicity that can accommodate such experience, and his interest in pre-modern and esoteric attempts to articulate these kinds of experience and concept already place his thought about disenchantment and its undoing beyond the pale for many commentators (Macey 2000: 212). Deleuze, however, would have been unlikely to reject Jung's thought for these reasons. For he too was interested in experiences or 'encounters' (1968a: 176) that shock common sense, in developing novel concepts based on such experiences, and in exploring what Hermeticism and related currents might have to offer modern thought (Kerslake 2007: 159–88; Ramey 2012). Nevertheless, within Jung's thinking about the whole there are several features, including ones associated with his esoteric sources, that reflect ideas Deleuze, in his thinking about the whole, did specifically target.

Deleuze was positive about the concept of the whole when, as in Henri Bergson's thought, it was conceived as something 'neither given nor giveable' (1983: 9), that is, as something that does not have a pregiven or fixed nature or static endpoint but is in a process of continual becoming and creativity. '[I]f the whole is not giveable', Deleuze maintained, 'it is because it is the Open, and because its nature is to change constantly, or to give rise to something new' (ibid.). He thus insisted that the whole not be confused with 'a closed set of objects' (ibid.).

The whole was, rather, 'that which prevents each set, however big it is, from closing in on itself, and that which forces it to extend itself into a larger set' (ibid.: 16).

It was against closed wholes that Deleuze levelled his criticism, in particular against formulations of the whole as either pre-existent or the goal of some future realisation, as organic in the sense that the whole governed and gave meaning to the parts of which it was composed, and as constituted by internal relations that determined its essence. In the 1972 revision of *Proust and Signs*, Deleuze contrasted two ways in which a fragment or sign could 'speak':

[A fragment or sign can speak] either because it permits us to divine the whole from which it is taken, to reconstitute the organism or the statue to which it belongs, and to seek out the other part that belongs to it – or else, on the contrary, because there is no other part that corresponds to it, no totality into which it can enter, no unity from which it is torn and to which it can be restored.

(Deleuze 1972: 112)

The former way reflects the view of the ancient Greeks as well as of Medieval and Renaissance Platonism (ibid.). The latter way reflects modernist literature such as Marcel Proust's *À la Recherche du Temps Perdu*, in which, wrote Deleuze, 'One would look in vain […] for platitudes about the work of art as an organic totality in which [as in holistic conceptions] each part predetermined the whole and in which the whole determines the part' (ibid.: 114). In the fragmented universe of Proust's novel, 'there is no Logos that gathers up all the pieces, hence no law attaches them to a whole to be regained or even formed' (ibid.: 131). For Deleuze, the whole is precisely the multiplicity of fragments – fragments that are related to one another only through 'sheer difference' and not through being parts of either an original or a future whole (Deleuze and Guattari 1972: 42). As Deleuze and his co-author Félix Guattari expressed it in *Anti-Oedipus*: 'We no longer believe in a primordial totality that once existed or in a final totality that awaits us at some future date'. Rather:

We believe only in totalities that are peripheral. And if we discover such a totality alongside various separate parts, it is a whole *of* these particular parts but does not totalise them; it is a unity *of* all of these particular parts but does not unify them; it is added to them as a new part fabricated separately.

(Deleuze and Guattari 1972: 42)

Earlier in this chapter I drew on a formal definition of holism (Phillips 1976) to demonstrate how closely Jung's thought fits with such definitions. The author of that definition, Denis Phillips, concluded that in holism as it has generally been understood in the social sciences, the kinds of relations of the parts of a whole both to the whole that they constitute and to one another are identical to the 'internal relations' theorised by neo-Hegelian thought (ibid.: 7–20). 'The parts of an organic [i.e., holistic] system are internally related to each other', writes Phillips (ibid.: 7), such that any change to the relations alters the parts and hence also the whole: in other words, 'entities are *necessarily* altered by the relations into which they enter' (ibid.: 8). As Patrick Hayden has clarified in a discussion of Deleuze's empiricism, this implies that systems and entities have essences from which their relations derive (Hayden 1995: 284–85). In the understanding of wholes affirmed by Deleuze, by contrast, relations are not derived from the essence of things or from their parts but are external to them, so that the relations can be changed without affecting the terms related (ibid.: 286). This leads to a view of entities and systems, including 'wholes', as not essences but constructions (ibid.: 286–87; see also Roffe 2010: 304–5).

The problem for Deleuze with the three interrelated notions of pre-existent (or original) and future (or restored) wholes, organicism, and internal relations was that they each presupposed and reinforced the idea of transcendence, that is, the idea that there is a level of reality separate from, superior to, and governing the empirical world. Pre-existent or future wholes imply beginning or end points outside the process of becoming, of which any experiential wholes are either degraded or not yet fully realised versions. They also imply determinism and finalism, both of which negate the openness and creativity of becoming.

No less problematically, organicism postulates a unity over and above and governing its organs or parts, with the subordinated parts drawing their meaning only from their function within the whole. Moreover, the organic view of wholes privileges individual living organisms over other forms of nature, such as the inorganic and the social (Protevi 2012: 248–49), thereby giving rise to an image of the whole of nature that in fact reflects only some of its forms. This was particularly problematic for Deleuze since, as John Protevi explains, he saw organisms as tending to assume 'habituated patterns' or 'strata', resulting in 'a centralised, hierarchical, and strongly patterned body' (2012: 257), which prevents the body from being 'open to new orderings and new potentials' (ibid.).

Finally, the notion of internal relations with its essentialist implications also, as Hayden explains, underpins a view of reality as 'an organic, stable, and absolute unity that transcends the empirical world […] a fixed Whole that transcends its parts', in contrast to Deleuze's preferred empiricist view, based on external relations, of reality as 'a series of shifting contingent wholes that form the immanent and open network of the world' (Hayden 1995: 286–87). The contrasting ethical, social, and political implications of these holistic and empiricist views that Deleuze respectively criticises and favours are well summarised by Hayden:

> On the one hand, essentialism and the paradigm of internal relations [i.e., organicistic holism] leads [sic] in the direction of extreme centralization and totalization, the subordination of individuals to transcendental principles, and passivity in the face of social and political homogeneity. On the other hand, pluralist empiricism and the theory and practice of external relations promotes [sic] decentralization and multiplicity, resistance to supposed universal necessities, and action with respect to the possibilities of creating new types of social and political association.
>
> (Hayden 1995: 287; see also Goodchild 2001: 158–59; Braidotti 2012; Patton 2012)

Organicistic holism in Jung

Where Deleuze condemned the notions of original and restored wholes, organicistic thinking, and internal relations because of their explicit and implicit appeals to transcendence, Jung arguably drew on all of these notions in support of his concept of wholeness. For example, he referred to 'the production and unfolding of the original, potential wholeness' (1917/1926/1943: §186); to 'the *a priori* existence of potential wholeness', on account of which, he stated, 'the idea of *entelechy* [a vital principle guiding an organism's or system's development and functioning] instantly recommends itself' (1951a: §278); and to an 'apocatastasis' or 'anamnesis' in which the 'ever-present archetype of wholeness', the 'original state of oneness with the God-image', would be restored (ibid.: §73; see also 1955–56: §§152, 660, 662). He described the *unus mundus*, with which the re-integrated mind-body is united in the third of Dorn's conjunctions, as 'the potential world of the first day of creation, when nothing was yet "in actu", i.e., divided into two and many, but was still one [...], the eternal Ground of all empirical being' (1955–56: §760).

Again, Jung included approvingly among the 'forerunners' of his deeply holistic concept of synchronicity (Main 2019) the Ancient Greek thinker Hippocrates and the Renaissance esoteric thinker Pico Della Mirandola, in both of whom organicism is explicit. For Hippocrates, as Jung quoted directly, 'all things are in sympathy. The whole organism and each one of its parts are working in conjunction for the same purpose' (in Jung 1952b: §924); while for Pico Della Mirandola, as Jung summarised, the world was 'one being, a visible God, in which everything is naturally arranged from the very beginning like the parts of a living organism' (Jung 1952b: §927). Jung's frequent references in his alchemical works to microcosm and macrocosm and notions of the 'Anthropos', 'Original Man', and 'Adam Kadmon' also imply an organicistic perspective (1944, 1951a, 1955–56).

It is less easy to find clear evidence of Jung's having been influenced by the notion of internal relations, as this is an idea stemming from philosophical traditions with which he did not directly engage. There are, however, indirect connections. The modern formulation of the idea of internal relations mainly derived from Hegel's philosophy of the Absolute (Phillips 1976: 7–20). As Glenn Magee has demonstrated, though, Hegel's own conception of the universe as an internally related whole was deeply influenced by the Hermetic notion that 'everything in the cosmos is internally related, bound up with everything else' (2001: 13–14). For Jung's part, even though he did not refer to the concept of internal relations as such, several of his ideas appear to suggest it: for example, his view of the mutual determination and dynamic interrelationship and interdependence of the self as the whole and the ego, shadow, and archetypes as its parts (Phillips 1976: 7–20; Main 2019: 61–63); and his statements, apropos synchronicity and the *unus mundus*, about 'the universal interrelationship of events' and 'an inter-connection and unity of causally unrelated [i.e., externally unrelated] events' (1955–56: §662).[4]

Finally, while Jung, like Deleuze, could express suspicion of the constricting and protective uses of transcendence – as when he charged the alchemists he otherwise so valued of having attempted to 'entrench themselves behind seemingly secure positions in the Beyond' with their 'metaphysical assertions' (1955–56: §680) – he nevertheless did not share Deleuze's zeal for rooting out transcendence entirely. On the contrary, he insisted that '[t]he concept of psychic wholeness necessarily involves an element of transcendence on account of the existence of unconscious components' (1958: §779). Again, after noting that 'the self can become a symbolic content of consciousness', he continued by also stressing that 'it is, as a superordinate totality, necessarily transcendental as well' (1951a: §264). And the final chapter of *Mysterium Coniunctionis*, while acknowledging the inevitable uncertainty of any representation of transcendental reality, nonetheless concludes by affirming that '[t]he existence of a transcendental reality is indeed evident in itself' and '[t]hat the world inside and outside ourselves rests on a transcendental background is as certain as our own existence' (1955–56: §787).

Prima facie, Jung's endorsement of the notions of original and restored wholes, organicistic thinking, internal relations, and transcendence suggests that his thought might be deeply vulnerable to a Deleuzian critique that would charge it with advocating a concept of the whole that intrinsically is static, promotes hierarchical and totalitarian relations intrapsychically, interpersonally, and culturally, and overall stymies creativity and open relationship. In the remainder of this chapter, I propose a perspective for thinking about Jung's and Deleuze's concepts of the whole, as well as of the relation between their bodies of thought more generally, from which this apparent vulnerability might be addressed.

Panentheism and the open whole

Christian McMillan, who has undertaken the most rigorous interrogation to date of the metaphysical logic and potential ethical dangers of

Jung's concept of the whole from a Deleuzian perspective (McMillan 2015), has identified some possible ways in which it could be argued, in response to the Deleuzian critique, that Jung's thought does after all support the idea of an open whole. One response would involve establishing connections between Jungian and Deleuzian thought in relation to contemporary scientific developments with which both thinkers can be aligned, such as in experimental physics, the philosophy of science, and the theory of emergence, where these fields promote the idea of open systems (ibid.: 21–25). Another response would be to focus on Jung's concept of synchronicity as providing a form of post-phenomenological access to the real through the 'shock' that synchronistic experiences give to normal thought and sensibility (ibid.: 21, 246–49). Other possible responses would involve reimagining some of Jung's more controversial concepts as ' "openings" to "enchanted Others" ' (McMillan 2018: 195) – concepts such as *esse in anima* (psychic reality), the psychoid, archetypes, and (again) synchronicity, each of which keeps the whole open by providing ways 'to think about the dynamic fluidity of [the] boundaries [of the psyche]' (ibid.). All of these responses would involve advancing a purely immanent interpretation of Jungian psychology.

The alternative response that I propose, rather than cast or recast Jung as a purely immanent thinker, queries the desirability and perhaps feasibility of eliminating transcendence. In anticipation, I distinguish between two different ways of understanding transcendence and argue that the kind of transcendence opposed by Deleuze was in fact also opposed by Jung, while the (different) kind of transcendence found in Jung is also discernible in Deleuze. From this perspective, Jung's and Deleuze's respective bodies of thought, including their ways of conceiving the whole, turn out to be quite close allies in challenging the first kind of transcendence, which arguably is what spawns both disenchantment and totalitarian thought.

Theism, pantheism, and panentheism

Deleuze's opposition to transcendence was epitomised by his assertion that 'the task of modern philosophy' was 'to overturn Platonism' (1968a: 71), with its subordination of sensible objects to intelligible (transcendent) ideas. The same opposition also drove his lifelong efforts to develop a philosophy of pure immanence (1968b, 2001), an aspiration expressed most blatantly in his admiration for Spinoza, whom he called the 'prince' and even the 'Christ' of philosophers because he 'never compromised with transcendence' but constructed a 'plane of immanence' that 'does not hand itself over to the transcendent, or restore any transcendence', thereby inspiring 'the fewest illusions, bad feelings, and erroneous perceptions' (Deleuze and Guattari 1991: 48, 60).

This alignment with Spinoza and aspiration towards pure immanence suggest that Deleuze's philosophy can be characterised as pantheistic (1968b: 333).[5] The definitive feature of pantheism is that it equates the divine with the world (nature, the cosmos), that is, it sees the divine as being no more than the world (Mander 2012; Buckareff and Nagasawa 2016: 2–3).[6] Among other things, this clearly implies that the divine is not separate from the world and is necessarily implicated in and affected by the world.

Pantheism strikingly contrasts with classical theism, such as underpins the mainstream religious thought of Judaism, Christianity, and Islam. In classical theism the divine is considered to be essentially separate from the world, to be unaffected by the world, and to be more than the world (Cooper 2006: 14–15; Buckareff and Nagasawa 2016: 1–2). It is against this conception of divine-world relations that Deleuze's criticisms of transcendence and alignment with pantheism appear to be levelled. For this classical theistic conception provides the pattern for relations where a separate eminent principle – the divine (or the one, or the mental) – is considered to be realer, more valuable, and regnant over that from which it is separated – the world (or the many, or the physical). Significantly, this same separation between the divine and the world was seen by Weber as the deep root of disenchantment (1904–5: 61, 178; Main 2017:1102–4).

However, pantheism is not the only way of conceiving the relationship between the divine and the world that would challenge classical theism. Akin to pantheism, but with a significant difference, is panentheism. Panentheism can be concisely defined as 'the belief or doctrine that God includes and interpenetrates the universe while being more than it' (*Shorter Oxford English Dictionary* 2002: 2080). Recognising that it comprises several varieties, Michael Brierley defines panentheism more fully but still generically in terms of the following three premises: 'First, that God is not separate from the cosmos [...]; second, that God is affected by the cosmos [...]; and third, that God is more than the cosmos' (2008: 639–40; see also Cooper 2006: 17–19; Buckareff and Nagasawa 2016: 2–3). Through the first two of Brierley's premises, panentheism is akin to pantheism, while through the third it differs. Specifically, panentheism affirms a kind of transcendence in that it considers the divine to be more than the world. But this transcendence differs from that of classical theism in that it expressly holds that the divine is not separate from the world and that the divine is affected by the world. Another way of expressing the differences between classical theism, pantheism, and panentheism would be to say that the relationship between the divine and the world in classical theism is chiefly characterised by transcendence, in pantheism is chiefly characterised by immanence, and in panentheism involves a balance between transcendence and immanence (cf. Asprem 2014: 281). As we shall now see, the perspective of panentheism could be a helpful framework for making sense of the tension we have uncovered between Jung's and Deleuze's respective concepts of the whole and their ethical implications.

Jung as an implicit panentheist

As I have argued in detail elsewhere (Main 2017: 1105–11), Jung's psychological model can be construed as underpinned by a form of implicit panentheism. This construal depends on Jung effectively having equated the unconscious with God: 'Recognising that [numinous experiences] do not spring from his conscious personality, [man] calls them mana, daimon, or God', Jung wrote, adding: 'Science employs the term "unconscious"' (1963: 368) – a position that is as much a sacralisation of psychology as it is a psychologisation of the sacred (cf. Hanegraaff 1998: 224–29). Jung's statements about God, or the God-image, in *Answer to Job* and elsewhere, depict God as not separate from the world, as affected by the world, and as more than the world (1952a: §§631, 686, 758); and correlatively his statements about the unconscious depict it as not separate from consciousness, as affected by consciousness, and as more than consciousness (1952a: §§538, 555, 557–58; 1963: 358; Main 2017: 1108–10).

Construing Jung's thought as panentheistic supports the characterisation of it at the beginning of this chapter, where it was shown to be holistic and to challenge the propositions underlying disenchantment. Thus, a recent study of Karl Christian Friedrich Krause (1781–1832), who coined the term 'panentheism' in the early nineteenth century, argues that Krause's concept not only anticipated recent thinking about holism but still provides an insightful theoretical framework for it (Göcke 2018: 196–200). Indeed, Brierley's generic definition of panentheism arguably could be applied to holism: that is, in holism the whole is not separate from the parts, is affected by the parts, and yet is more than the parts. With regard to disenchantment, I have detailed in a previous publication how the metaphysical logic of panentheism undoes each of the defining features of this condition, using Jung's thought as an illustration (Main 2017). And it is worth noting that Western esotericism, perhaps the most literal carrier of enchantment as well as one of the deep cultural influences on holistic thought (Hanegraaff 1998; Dusek 1999: 99–205) and a major source for Jung, has in its turn been convincingly shown to be based on panentheistic thought (Magee 2001: 8–9; Hanegraaff 2012: 371; Asprem 2014: 77–79, 279–84).

Even more pertinently, however, construing Jung's thought as panentheistic shows how his concept of the whole, together with the involved notions of original and restored wholes, organicism, and internal relations, might remain open and not after all be vulnerable to the Deleuzian critique. If Jung's concept of the whole, that is, the self, is both transcendent and immanent, it both exceeds the possibility of being completely expressed (insofar as it is an archetype in itself) and receives an ongoing multiplicity of necessarily partial empirical expressions (archetypal images). The dynamic between the transcendence and immanence here keeps the concept open by ensuring that, while the archetypal images express ever-different aspects or formulations of wholeness, no archetypal image is a final or complete expression of the whole. Each image gives an approximate expression that resolves the tensions and problems being experienced at the time, but that resolution, as now a conscious image, itself immediately and recursively becomes part of a new set of tensions and problems, which in turn requires resolution through the emergence of another archetypal image. In other words, the transcendent aspect of the whole is kept from being static by its non-separation from and ability to be affected by the world of becoming; while the immanent aspect of the whole is kept from being static by being continually destabilised by the 'more' of the transcendent.

Jung's openness to such a dynamic concept of transcendence, where the transcendent is envisaged as implicated with becoming, can be seen when he states at the beginning of 'Answer to Job' that 'we can imagine God as *an eternally flowing current of vital energy that endlessly changes shape* just as easily as we can imagine him as an eternally unmoved, unchangeable essence' (1952a: §555, emphasis added). More empirically, his recognition that even the most stable, symmetrical, and ordered symbols of wholeness are necessarily subject to continual change was expressed in his observation that the mandala – the paramount symbol of the self (1963: 221) and the 'empirical equivalent' of the *unus mundus* (1955–56: §661) – transforms from one manifestation to the next (1944: §§122–331; 1963: 220–22). As he wrote, citing Part Two of Goethe's *Faust*: 'Only gradually did I discover what the mandala really is: "Formation, Transformation, Eternal Mind's eternal recreation"' (1963: 221).

As well as keeping open his overall concept of the whole, the mutual implication of transcendence and immanence in Jung's panentheistic thought similarly ensures that his conceptions of original and restored wholes, organicism, and internal relations remain open. For example, in his statements about the restoration of an original wholeness (apocatastasis), Jung described the self as a state of 'potential wholeness' (1917/1926/1943: §186; 1951a: §278) and the *unus mundus* as 'the potential world of the first day of creation' (1955–56: §760). But what it means to realise this state or world of potential is to achieve 'a synthesis of the [immanent] conscious with the [transcendent] unconscious' (ibid.: §770), that is, a synthesis in which empirical consciousness reconnects with and becomes able more fully to express the *unus mundus* as a source of open-ended creativity. Again, insofar as Jung's statements about organicism and microcosm–macrocosm relations refer, directly or indirectly, to symbols of the self (such as the Hermetic notion of the 'Anthropos' and its synonyms), then this organicism and the related notion of microcosm–macrocosm are no more promoting a closed system than is the concept of the self. Finally, any version of internal relations that can be found in Jung's work is similarly not closed, for the 'universal interrelationship of events' (1955–56: §661) postulated by Jung on the basis of synchronicity accords with what 'can be verified empirically' (1952b: §938). It is a potential but contingent and open relationship that, by transgressing normal spatiotemporal and psychophysical limits, can connect even the most distant and divergent events (ibid.: §840). But it is explicitly not, as in Leibniz, for example, 'a complete pre-established parallelism' expressing an 'absolute rule' (ibid.: §938). In a statement with relevance for the influence on him of pre-modern and esoteric thought generally, Jung described synchronicity as 'a *modern differentiation* of the obsolete concept of correspondence, sympathy, and harmony' (1951b: §995; emphasis added). It was a 'modern differentiation' precisely by virtue of being based on 'empirical experience and experimentation' (ibid.).

Deleuze as an implicit panentheist

As well as helping to make sense of how Jung's thought, despite its appeals to transcendence, can remain open, creative, and relational, the metaphysical logic of panentheism can help in resolving some difficulties that attach to Deleuze's attempt to articulate a philosophy of pure immanence. While Deleuze's efforts to root out all trace of transcendence from his philosophy have been found compelling and helpful by some commentators (e.g., Albert 2001; Ansell-Pearson 2001; Adkins 2018), others have found reasons to question this project. Alain Badiou, for example, has argued that Deleuze, with his 'metaphysics of the One' (2000: 10), far from reversing Platonism, himself establishes a 'Platonism of the virtual' (ibid.: 45). Phillip Goodchild has noted that, paradoxically, Deleuze's 'plane of immanence', as well as being transcend*al* in the Kantian sense of being 'a presupposition about the nature of thought', is also transcend*ent* in the Kantian sense inasmuch as it is 'a matter of being' (2001: 158). Again, Peter Hallward, while acknowledging that Deleuze's 'affirmation of absolute and immanent creativity certainly blocks any invocation of a transcendent "creator"', has suggested that this comes at the ethical and political cost of implying 'a philosophy that seeks to escape any mediation through the categories of subjectivity, history and the world' (2006: 3). And

Christopher Simpson has argued that the extreme form of transcendence opposed by Deleuze is a caricature – 'God as a static, univocal eternity – absolute in its immutability and stasis beyond time and becoming, and so unable to relate to the world' (2012: 78) – and that it is this caricature that generates the problematic 'dualism between God and the world' (ibid.) that Deleuze finds so objectionable. Like Badiou, Simpson also finds that Deleuze himself effectively reintroduced a form of transcendence through his concept of the virtual:

> Deleuze's actual and virtual are both real, but the virtual [...] is ultimately more real, the '"good" transcendental creative factor' having a definite privilege and priority over the '"bad" static and representable created element', over 'the illusory solidity of the actual'. In this way Deleuze's reversal of Platonism yet reflects a neo-Platonic or Gnostic dualism.
>
> (Simpson 2012: 79, quoting Justaert 2009: 542–43)

The weight of these criticisms of Deleuze's understanding of transcendence is certainly debatable, but one way in which they could be eased would be to see his thought as involving not a theistic but a panentheistic form of transcendence. The principal ground for making this move is that the same set of logical relationships that is found between the divine and the world in panentheism, and between the unconscious and consciousness in Jung's thought, can be found between the virtual and the actual in Deleuze's thought. The virtual (a field of potentiality comprising a multiplicity of 'problematic ideas') and the actual (specific occurrences representing the solutions to problematic ideas) are the two main characterisations of reality in Deleuze, and they reciprocally determine each other in an open-ended process of creativity (1968a: 214–74). Thus, for Deleuze, the virtual is not separate from the actual, since both are aspects of the same reality (ibid.: 260–61, 350); is affected by the actual, through 'a double process of reciprocal determination' (ibid.: 260; cf. the reference to 'counter-actualisation' below); and is more than the actual, inasmuch as the actual does not resemble and cannot fully express the virtual (ibid.: 260–1, 264).[7]

That this construal of Deleuze's thought may not be entirely unwarranted is suggested by the helpful perspective on his views of transcendence offered by James Williams (2010) and Kristien Justaert (2012), both, significantly, drawing on the process philosophy of Alfred North Whitehead. In language reminiscent of Deleuze, Whitehead had written about how '[t]he vicious separation of the flux from the permanence leads to the concept of an entirely static God, with eminent reality, in relation to an entirely fluent world, with deficient reality' (1929: 346). Yet Whitehead did not, as Deleuze did, aim to resolve this separation by eliminating transcendence and advocating pure immanence. As Williams explicates:

> For Whitehead, separated transcendence is pure stasis, meaningless because no change whatsoever can take place within it, a timeless and momentum free block. Yet pure immanence is equally nonsensical, since as pure flux we cannot explain its valued forward momentum and novelty, it becomes free of any realities and without sense.
>
> (Williams 2010: 98)

Whitehead conceived of the divine as dipolar, having both a transcendent 'primordial nature' and an immanent 'consequent nature' (1929: 31, 343–45). Williams explains that the two movements stemming from these two natures correspond to the two co-existing movements described by Deleuze as explication and complication (Williams 2010: 102; see Deleuze 1968b: 175–76), and he suggests that the relations resulting from the two movements for Whitehead precisely match Deleuze's description: '*The multiple is in the one* which complicates it, as much as *the one is in the multiple* that explains it' (Deleuze 2003: 244, quoted in Williams 2010: 101; Williams's emphasis). Put in terms of Deleuze's alternative vocabulary of the virtual and the actual, this is to say that the actual is in the virtual and the virtual is in the actual. Just as for Whitehead's metaphysics there is a 'creative circle moving from abstract eternal realm through a creative transformation in the actual and back to a now transformed virtual real', so in Deleuze's thought, as expressed for example in *Logic of Sense* (Deleuze 1969: 149–51), 'Ideas or sense move through surface or intensity to an actual realm, where a counter-actualisation reworks the form and power of the virtual, sending it back to return again as new creativity' (Williams 2010: 96). In terms echoing characterisations of panentheism, Williams concludes that 'Deleuze's work is open to an interpretation where immanence and transcendence are never treated as fully separable, but rather must be considered as essentially and indivisibly related as processes' (2010: 102; cf. Ramey 2012: 207). Justaert makes this complex set of relationships even more explicit:

> In Whitehead's philosophical system, the actual (God's consequent nature or the many) influences and even changes the virtual (God's primordial nature or the one); and while the primordial nature of God is a form of pure potentiality for Whitehead, his consequent nature is both physical and actual. The actual therefore ensures that the virtual does not become a static transcendence. Indeed, there are continuous fluxes and becomings between the two ways of being. 'It is as true to say that God creates the World, as that the World creates God', Whitehead concludes.
>
> (Justaert 2012: 77, quoting Whitehead 1929: 348)

Whitehead was one of the twentieth-century philosophers whom Deleuze most revered.[8] Yet, far from eschewing the notions of organicism and internal relations, Whitehead considered these notions integral to how he understood the nature of reality as process: he referred to his philosophy as 'the philosophy of organism' (1929: 18 *et passim*) and he invoked internal relations, not just external relations, to make sense of the 'actual occasions' that he considered to be the basic units of reality (ibid.: 308–9). Although, like Jung, he did not appear to be aware of the concept of panentheism, his reflections on 'God and the World' at the conclusion of *Process and Reality* have been foundational for process panentheism, one of the most prominent currents of contemporary panentheistic thought (Cooper 2006: 165–93). Together these features of Whitehead's philosophy suggest, *pace* Deleuze, that the notions of transcendence, original and restored wholes, organicism, and internal relations can be understood in ways compatible with a rigorously articulated philosophy of becoming and process. In turn, this makes plausible the suggestion that Deleuze's own philosophy could be productively construed as panentheistic.

The more widely held view of Deleuze appears to be that, although his work involves 'a certain thought of unity', nevertheless 'we cannot consider him to be a "holist" in any direct sense' (Roffe 2010: 305).

In light of the above panentheistic considerations, however, Justaert would disagree:

> Deleuze's (and even Spinoza's) metaphysics reflects a holistic and monistic view of creation: the One (God/Being) and the many (creation/beings) are two sides of the same coin. They are related to each other through the act of expression. God expresses Himself in the whole of creation in the same way.
>
> (Justaert 2012: 30)

Conclusion

From the perspective of a panentheistic metaphysics, it appears that Jung's holistic thought can escape the kinds of criticism that Deleuze levelled against forms of transcendence that foster totalitarianism. Such problematic forms of transcendence stem from a theistic metaphysics, which considers there to be an essential separation between the divine and the world. However, the form of transcendence that can be found in Jung and that informed his explicit and implicit use of the notions of original and restored wholes, organicism, and internal relations was panentheistic and as such denied any essential separation between the divine and the world. Arguably, Jung was as opposed as was Deleuze to theistic transcendence, for it was the divine-world separation of theistic transcendence that also spawned the condition of disenchantment against which so much of Jung's own critical energy was exerted (Main 2017: 1102–4). In the end, Deleuze and Jung appear to have shared a common critical target in theistic transcendence.

The case of Jung's psychology thus suggests that at least some influential forms of holistic thought have no intrinsic relationship to totalitarianism. Indeed, Jung's psychology even provides an example of how holistic thought can be deployed as a prophylactic against totalitarian thought, as when Jung argued in 'The undiscovered self' that realisation of the wholeness of the self through individuation can serve, as religion had once done, as a counterbalance to the mass-mindedness out of which totalitarianism was prone to emerge (1957; see also McMillan 2021).

The holism that Jung promoted centres on a concept, the self, which involves a synthesis of (immanent) ego-consciousness with the (transcendent) unconscious. This involvement of the unconscious ensures that the concept of the whole informing conscious thought remains in a process of transformation, open to ever-new possibilities of connection and creation. For Jung it was one-sided and fixated ego-consciousness rather than the self that was associated with the problematic forms of despotic thought traced by Deleuze to transcendence. This is evident from Jung's comments about the 'new ethic' that Erich Neumann identified as implied by the depth psychological aim of uniting consciousness and the unconscious in the individuation process:

> [Neumann] compares the relation to the unconscious with a parliamentary democracy, whereas the old ethic [a collective morality based on ethical rules] unconsciously imitates, or actually prefers, the procedure of an absolute monarchy or a tyrannical one-party system. Through the new ethic, the ego-consciousness is ousted from its central position in a psyche organized on the lines of a monarchy or totalitarian state, its place being taken by *wholeness* or the *self*, which is now recognized as central.
>
> (Jung 1949: §1419)

If there are problematic associations of Jung's thought with totalitarian currents of his day, these, such as they may be, would appear to exist despite rather than because of the structure of his thought, and need to be examined historically and biographically.

This said, there is scarcely ground for complacency. For it is possible for ego-consciousness to fall out of relationship with the unconscious at any point, especially when, as is often and even typically the case, the confrontation of ego-consciousness with the unconscious is painful or otherwise difficult. At that point, the integration so far achieved by ego-consciousness could indeed become defensively fixed and thereby provide the basis for the development of totalitarian formations. Awareness of this possibility, sharpened by the confrontation with Deleuzian thought, adds urgency to the task of maintaining the relationship between ego-consciousness and the unconscious, which for Jung would mean persisting vigilantly in the lifelong process of individuation.

For Deleuze's philosophy, in its turn, the confrontation with Jung's thought, in particular the suggestion that has emerged that Deleuze could also be understood as an implicit panentheist, might help to reframe some of the problems that certain scholars have found with his understanding of transcendence and his attempt to articulate a philosophy of pure immanence. Finally, viewing Deleuze as an implicit panentheist could also provide a context within which some of Deleuze's important, but in his own writings less foregrounded, influences could emerge more fully into view, including those of Western esotericism, Whitehead, and not least Jung.

Acknowledgement

Work on this chapter was supported by the Arts and Humanities Research Council [AH/N003853/1].

Notes

1 For a detailed discussion of the issues involved in defining holism, see Main, McMillan, and Henderson (2020).
2 In view of Popper's explicit criticism of the alleged totalitarian implications of holism, his philosophical perspective might have been an alternative one to use for confronting Jung. However, the holism that Popper criticises is specifically social holism – the view that social entities have properties that are irreducible to the behaviours of the individuals composing those social entities – and Jung, while seemingly a thoroughgoing holist in relation to the development of individuals, was himself critical of social holism (1957, §§504, 553–54). In their study of medical holism between 1920 and 1950 Christopher Lawrence and George Weisz (1998) observe that 'there have been two rather different holistic responses to modernity', one emphasising 'the need for *individual* wholeness, plenitude, or authenticity' and the other 'the submergence of the individual within a larger entity — nation, race, religious community, nature' (1998: 7). Popper's target was the latter response. Jung's holism concerns itself with the former.
3 The term 'holism' was not coined until 1926 and appeared in a work written in English (Smuts 1926). Jung, like many other German-speaking intellectuals, continued to use the established term *Ganzheit* and its cognates (*Ganzheitlichkeit*, etc.) rather than *Holismus*, the derived German form of the English neologism.
4 Sean Kelly draws detailed parallels between Jung's concept of the self and Hegel's concept of the Absolute in a study centring on the two thinkers' shared implicit notion of 'complex holism' (Kelly 1993). While Kelly does

not himself foreground the concept of internal relations, his study arguably provides a basis for doing so.

5 Deleuze himself characterised his thought, along with Spinoza's, as atheistic (Deleuze and Guattari 1991: 92). This does not necessarily contradict their characterisation as pantheistic. Since the eighteenth century, pantheism has often been charged with being equivalent to atheism, inasmuch as the pantheistic denial of any distinction between God and the world can seem to do away with the need for any separate discourse about God. Furthermore, in one sense pantheism certainly is 'a-theistic' in that it negates classical theism. However, neither Deleuze nor Spinoza would have approved a form of atheism that denied the sacredness of the world or the role of the infinite within it. They aimed not to banish the divine from their thought but to locate, or re-locate, it entirely within the world (nature, cosmos), if not as the world.

6 There are, of course, multiple ways of understanding pantheism, theism, and panentheism and the borders between them are often difficult to determine. For the purpose of setting out my broad argument in what follows, it has seemed sufficient, as well as practical, to adopt quite wide, generic definitions of the terms.

7 Also suggestive of panentheism is Deleuze's formulation that '[t]he problem is at once both transcendent and immanent in relation to its solutions' (1968a: 203).

8 For further discussion of the relationship between Deleuze and Whitehead, see Robinson (2009).

References

(In the citations and reference list, dates within parentheses refer to the date of original publication. The date of edition consulted, if different, appears after the publisher in the reference list.)

Adkins, B. (2018). To have done with the transcendental: Deleuze, immanence, intensity. *Journal of Speculative Philosophy 32*(3): 533–43.

Albert, E. (2001). Deleuze's impersonal, hylozoic cosmology: The expulsion of theology. In M. Bryden (Ed.), *Deleuze and Religion*, 184–95. London and New York: Routledge.

Ansell-Pearson, K. (2001). Pure reserve: Deleuze, philosophy, and immanence. In M. Bryden (Ed.), *Deleuze and Religion*, 141–55. London and New York: Routledge.

Ansell-Pearson, K. (2007). Beyond the human condition: An introduction to Deleuze's lecture course. *SubStance #114 36*(3): 1–15.

Asprem, E. (2014). *The Problem of Disenchantment: Scientific Naturalism and Esoteric Discourse 1900–1939*. Leiden: Brill.

Badiou, A. (2000). *Deleuze: The Clamor of Being* (L. Churchill, Trans.). Minneapolis, MN: University of Minnesota Press.

Berman, M. (1981). *The Reenchantment of the World*. Ithaca, NY: Cornell University Press.

Braidotti, R. (2012). Nomadic ethics. In D. Smith and H. Somers-Hall (Eds.), *The Cambridge Companion to Deleuze*, 170–97. Cambridge: Cambridge University Press.

Brierley, M. (2008). The potential of panentheism for dialogue between science and religion. In P. Clayton and Z. Simpson (Eds.), *The Oxford Handbook of Religion and Science*, 635–51. Oxford: Oxford University Press.

Buckareff, A., and Nagasawa, Y. (2016). Introduction: Alternative conceptions of divinity and contemporary analytic philosophy of religion. In A. Buckareff and Y. Nagasawa (Eds.), *Alternative Concepts of God: Essays on the Metaphysics of the Divine*, 1–20. Oxford: Oxford University Press.

Cambray, J. (2009). *Synchronicity: Nature and Psyche in an Interconnected Universe*. College Station, TX: Texas A&M University Press.

Cooper, D. (1996). *Verstehen*, holism and fascism. *Royal Institute of Philosophy Supplement 41*: 95–107.

Cooper, J. (2006). *Panentheism: The Other God of the Philosophers: From Plato to the present*. Nottingham, UK: Apollos.

Deleuze, G. (1968a). *Difference and Repetition* (P. Patton, Trans.). London: Bloomsbury, 2014.

Deleuze, G. (1968b). *Expressionism in Philosophy: Spinoza* (M. Joughin, Trans.). New York: Zone, 2013.

Deleuze, G. (1969). *The Logic of Sense* (C. Boundas, Ed.; M. Lester and C. Stivale, Trans.). New York: Columbia University Press, 1990.

Deleuze, G. (1972). *Proust and Signs: The Complete Text* (R. Howard, Trans.). London: Athlone, 2000; original French publication 1964).

Deleuze, G. (1983). *Cinema 1: The Movement-Image* (H. Tomlinson and B. Habberjam, Trans.). London: Athlone Press, 1992.

Deleuze, G. (2001). *Pure Immanence: Essays on A Life*. New York: Zone.

Deleuze, G. (2003). Les plages d'immanence. In D. Lapoujade (Ed.), *Deux Régimes de Fous*, 244–46. Paris: Seuil.

Deleuze, G., and Guattari, F. (1972). *Anti-Oedipus: Capitalism and Schizophrenia* (R. Hurley, M. Seem, and H. Lane, Trans.). Minneapolis, MN: University of Minnesota Press, 2000.

Deleuze, G., and Guattari, F. (1991). *What is Philosophy?* (H Tomlinson and G. Burchell, Trans.). New York: Columbia University Press, 1994.

Dusek, V. (1999). *The Holistic Inspirations of Physics: The Underground History of Electromagnetic Theory*. New Brunswick, NJ: Rutgers University Press.

Esfeld, M. (2003). Philosophical holism. In *Encyclopedia of Life Support Systems*. Paris: UNESCO/Eolss Publishers [www.eolss.net].

Fellows, A. (2019). *Gaia, Psyche and Deep Ecology: Navigating Climate Change in the Anthropocene*. London and New York: Routledge.

Göcke, B. (2018). *The Panentheism of Karl Christian Friedrich Krause (1781–1832): From Transcendental Philosophy to Metaphysics*. Berlin: Peter Lang.

Goodchild. P. (2001). Why is philosophy so compromised with God? In M. Bryden (Ed.), *Deleuze and Religion*, 156–166. London and New York: Routledge.

Grossman, S. (1979). C. G. Jung and National Socialism. *Journal of European Studies 9*: 231–59.

Hallward, P. (2006). *Out of This World: Deleuze and the Philosophy of Creation*. London and New York: Verso.

Hanegraaff, W. (1998). *New Age Religion and Western Culture: Esotericism in the Mirror of Secular Thought*. Albany, NY: State University of New York Press.

Hanegraaff, W. (2012). *Esotericism and the Academy: Rejected Knowledge in Western Culture*. Cambridge: Cambridge University Press.

Harrington, A. (1996). *Reenchanted Science: Holism in German Culture from Wilhelm II to Hitler*. Princeton, NJ: Princeton University Press.

Hayden, P. (1995). From relations to practice in the empiricism of Gilles Deleuze. *Man and World 28*: 283–302.

Heelas, P., and Woodhead, L, with B. Seel, B. Szeszynski, and K. Tusting (2005). *The Spiritual Revolution: Why Religion is Giving Way to Spirituality*. Oxford: Blackwell.

Holland, E. (2012). Deleuze and psychoanalysis. In D. Smith and H. Somers-Hall (Eds.), *The Cambridge Companion to Deleuze*, 307–36. Cambridge: Cambridge University Press.

Jung, C. G. (1911–12/1952). *The Collected Works of C. G. Jung* (Sir H. Read, M. Fordham, and G. Adler, Eds.; W. McGuire, Exec. Ed.; R. F. C. Hull, Trans.) [hereafter *Collected Works*], vol. 5, *Symbols of Transformation*, 2nd ed. London: Routledge and Kegan Paul, 1967.

Jung, C. G. (1917/1926/1943). On the psychology of the unconscious. In *Collected Works*, vol. 7, *Two Essays on Analytical Psychology*, 2nd ed., 1–119. London: Routledge and Kegan Paul, 1966.

Jung, C. G. (1921). *Collected Works*, vol. 6, *Psychological Types*. London: Routledge and Kegan Paul, 1971.

Jung, C. G. (1928). The relations between the ego and the unconscious. In *Collected Works*, vol. 7, *Two Essays on Analytical Psychology*, 2nd ed., 121–241. London: Routledge and Kegan Paul, 1966.

Jung, C. G. (1937). Psychological factors in human behaviour. In *Collected Works*, vol. 8, *The Structure and Dynamics of the Psyche*, 2nd ed., 114–25. London: Routledge and Kegan Paul, 1969.

Jung, C. G. (1940). The psychology of the child archetype. In *Collected Works*, vol. 9i, *The Archetypes and the Collective Unconscious*, 2nd ed., 149–81. London: Routledge and Kegan Paul, 1968.

Jung, C. G. (1944). *Collected Works*, vol. 12, *Psychology and Alchemy*, 2nd ed. London: Routledge and Kegan Paul, 1968.

Jung, C. G. (1945). Psychotherapy today. In *Collected Works*, vol. 16, *The Practice of Psychotherapy*, 2nd ed., 94–110. London: Routledge and Kegan Paul, 1966.

Jung, C. G. (1946). The psychology of the transference. In *Collected Works*, vol. 16, *The Practice of Psychotherapy*, 2nd ed., 163–323. London: Routledge and Kegan Paul, 1966.

Jung, C. G. (1947/1954). On the nature of the psyche. In *Collected Works*, vol. 8, *The Structure and Dynamics of the Psyche*, 2nd ed., 159–234. London: Routledge and Kegan Paul, 1969.

Jung, C. G. (1949). Foreword to Neumann: 'Depth psychology and a new ethic'. In *Collected Works*, vol. 18, *The Symbolic Life*, 616–22. London: Routledge and Kegan Paul, 1977.

Jung, C. G. (1951a). *Collected Works*, vol. 9ii, *Aion*, 2nd ed. London: Routledge and Kegan Paul, 1968.

Jung, C. G. (1951b). On synchronicity. In *Collected Works*, vol. 8, *The Structure and Dynamics of the Psyche*, 2nd ed., 520–31. London: Routledge and Kegan Paul, 1969.

Jung, C. G. (1952a). Answer to Job. In *Collected Works*, vol. 11, *Psychology and Religion: West and East*, 2nd ed., 355–470. London: Routledge and Kegan Paul, 1969.

Jung, C. G. (1952b). Synchronicity: An acausal connecting principle. In *Collected Works*, vol. 8, *The Structure and Dynamics of the Psyche*, 2nd ed., 417–519. London: Routledge and Kegan Paul, 1969.

Jung, C. G. (1955–56). *Collected Works*, vol. 14, *Mysterium Coniunctionis: An Inquiry into the Separation and Synthesis of Psychic Opposites in Alchemy*, 2nd ed. London: Routledge and Kegan Paul, 1970.

Jung, C. G. (1957). The undiscovered self (Present and future). In *Collected Works*, vol. 10, *Civilization in Transition*, 2nd ed., 245–305. London: Routledge and Kegan Paul, 1970.

Jung, C. G. (1958). Flying saucers: A modern myth of things seen in the skies. In *Collected Works*, vol. 10, *Civilization in Transition*, 2nd ed., 307–433. London: Routledge and Kegan Paul, 1970.

Jung, C. G. (1963). *Memories, Dreams, Reflections* (A. Jaffé, Ed.; R. and C. Winston, Trans.). London: Fontana, 1995.

Justaert, K. (2009). Gilles Deleuze: Évaluation théologique. *Laval Théologique et Philosophique 65*(3): 531–44.

Justaert, K. (2012). *Theology After Deleuze*. London: Continuum.

Kelly, S. (1993). *Individuation and the Absolute: Hegel, Jung and the Path Toward Wholeness*. New York: Paulist Press.

Kerslake, C. (2007). *Deleuze and the Unconscious*. London: Continuum.

Keulartz, J. (1998). *The Struggle for Nature: A Critique of Radical Ecology* (R. Kuitenbrouwer, Trans.). London: Routledge.

Lawrence, C., and Weisz, G. (Eds.) (1998). *Greater than the Parts: Holism in Biomedicine 1920–1950*. Oxford: Oxford University Press.

Macey, D. (Ed.) (2000). *The Penguin Dictionary of Critical Theory*. London: Penguin.

Magee, G. A. (2001). *Hegel and the Hermetic Tradition*. Ithaca, NY: Cornell University Press.

Maidenbaum, A., and Martin, S. (1992). *Lingering Shadows: Jungians, Freudians and Anti-Semitism*. Boston, MA: Shambhala.

Main, R. (2011). Synchronicity and the limits of re-enchantment. *International Journal of Jungian Studies 3*(2): 144–58.

Main, R. (2013). Myth, synchronicity, and re-enchantment. In L. Burnett, S. Bahun, and R. Main (Eds.), *Myth, Literature, and the Unconscious*, 129–46. London: Karnac.

Main, R. (2017). Panentheism and the undoing of disenchantment. *Zygon: Journal of Religion and Science 52*(4): 1098–122.

Main, R. (2019). Synchronicity and holism. In *Analytical Psychology Meets Academic Research: Avignon Conference 2018*, 59–74. *Revue de Psychologie Analytique* (Hors série).

Main, R., McMillan, C., and Henderson, D. (2020). Introduction. In C. McMillan, R. Main, and D. Henderson (Eds.), *Holism: Possibilities and Problems*, 1–14. London and New York: Routledge.

Mander, W. (2012). Pantheism. In E. Zalta (Ed.), *The Stanford Encyclopedia of Philosophy* (Winter 2016 Edition) [https://plato.stanford.edu/archives/win2016/entries/pantheism/].

McMillan, C. (2015). The 'image of thought' in Jung's 'Whole-Self': A critique. Unpublished PhD thesis, University of Essex, UK.

McMillan, C. (2018). Jung and Deleuze: Enchanted openings to the Other: A philosophical contribution. *International Journal of Jungian Studies 10*(3): 184–98.

McMillan, C. (2021). The 'image of thought' and the State-form in Jung's 'The undiscovered self' and Deleuze and Guattari's 'Treatise on nomadology'. In

R. Main, C. McMillan, and D. Henderson (Eds.). *Jung, Deleuze, and the Problematic Whole*. London and New York: Routledge.

Papadopoulos, R. (2006). Jung's epistemology and methodology. In R. Papadopoulos (Ed.), *The Handbook of Jungian Psychology: Theory, Practice and Applications*, 5–53. London and New York: Routledge.

Patton, P. (2012). Deleuze's political philosophy. In D. Smith and H. Somers-Hall (Eds.), *The Cambridge Companion to Deleuze*, 198–219. Cambridge: Cambridge University Press.

Phillips, D. C. (1976). *Holistic Thought in Social Science*. Stanford, CA: Stanford University Press.

Popper, K. (1945). *The Open Society and Its Enemies*. London: Routledge and Kegan Paul.

Popper, K. (1957). *The Poverty of Historicism*. London: Routledge and Kegan Paul.

Protevi, J. (2012). Deleuze and life. In D. Smith and H. Somers-Hall (Eds.), *The Cambridge Companion to Deleuze*, 239–64. Cambridge: Cambridge University Press.

Ramey, J. (2012). *The Hermetic Deleuze: Philosophy and Spiritual Ordeal*. Durham, NC: Duke University Press.

Robinson, K. (Ed.) (2009). *Deleuze, Whitehead, Bergson: Rhizomatic Connections*. Basingstoke, UK: Palgrave Macmillan.

Roffe, J. (2010). Whole. In A. Parr (Ed.), *The Deleuze Dictionary*, rev. ed., 304–5. Edinburgh: Edinburgh University Press.

Shorter Oxford English Dictionary (2002). 5th ed. (W. Trumble and A. Stevenson, Eds.). Oxford: Oxford University Press.

Simpson, C. (2012). *Deleuze and Theology*. London: Bloomsbury/T & T Clark.

Smith, C. (1990). *Jung's Quest for Wholeness: A Religious and Historical Perspective*. Albany, NY: State University of New York Press.

Smuts, J. (1926). *Holism and Evolution*. London: Macmillan.

Weber, M. (1904–5). *The Protestant Ethic and the Spirit of Capitalism*. London: Routledge, 2001.

Weber, M. (1919). Science as a vocation. In Hans H. Gerth and C. Wright Mills (Eds.), *From Max Weber: Essays in Sociology*, 129–55. New York: Oxford University Press.

Whitehead, A. N. (1929). *Process and Reality: Corrected Edition* (D. Griffin and D. Sherburne, Eds.). London and New York: Macmillan, 1979.

Williams, J. (2010). Immanence and transcendence as inseparable processes: On the relevance of arguments from Whitehead to Deleuze interpretation. *Deleuze Studies* 4(1): 94–106.

Chapter 2

The 'image of thought' and the State-form in Jung's 'The undiscovered self' and Deleuze and Guattari's 'Treatise on nomadology'

Christian McMillan

Introduction

This chapter focuses on a number of conceptual affinities that appear within the work of Swiss depth psychologist C. G. Jung (1875–1961) and the work of French philosopher Gilles Deleuze (1925–1995) and his co-writer Félix Guattari (1930–1992). I draw extensively from one of Jung's final essays, 'The undiscovered self (present and future)' (1957), which was first published after both world wars and just after the period of the Red Scare in the United States. Jung's essay is noteworthy for its critical exigencies on the role of the State[1] in modern times. Jung analyses the ways in which the State organises and orientates thought in a certain one-sided manner. He considers the negative logical and ethical effects of this organisation on the individual, religion, and science. When in conformity with the State, these three systems reinforce the way in which the State organises and orientates an image of thought whose effects serve to exclude alternative forms of organisation.

In 'The undiscovered self' Jung presents arguments that attest to the psychological causes and consequences of the organisation of thought when it is universalised by the State. Likewise, Deleuze tends to focus on the organisation and distribution of relations within thought systems of which the State is one variation (others include the organism, language, psychoanalysis, art, science, and religion). In the first half of the chapter, I examine concepts that Jung presents in his essay. Jung introduces positive concepts such as 'individual' and the 'whole man' and negative ones such as the 'mass man', 'statistical man' and the 'State'. Jung's positive concepts can be read as gesturing to an alternative form of relations which share some affinities with Deleuze and

Guattari's affirmative characterisation of 'relations of exteriority' (the 'form of exteriority'). These characterisations feature alongside their critique of the 'State-form' from '1227: Treatise on nomadology – the war machine', which comprises the twelfth plateau of *A Thousand Plateaus: Capitalism and Schizophrenia* (1980/1987), a work they co-authored in 1980.

In the second half of the chapter, I consider Jung's analysis of the ways in which thought is orientated by the abstract idea of the State in modernity. I then relate this to Deleuze's critique of the image of thought which formed a crucial part of his *Difference and Repetition* (1968). I draw attention to the notion of the 'private thinker' that was first illuminated by Deleuze in *Difference and Repetition* and to which he returned in the 'Treatise on nomadology'. In this section I will argue that Jung's intentions in his essay exhibit many features which one can find in common with Deleuze and Guattari's notion of the 'private thinker', a 'thinker' capable of resisting a hegemonic and one-sided image of thought. This argument involves an engagement with Jung's conceptualisation of estranging encounters with the extramundane from 'The undiscovered self'. I argue that these encounters make possible a re-orientation of a one-sided image of thought. In the latter sections of this chapter, I consider these encounters in relation to Deleuze's emphasis on the role of 'the encounter', which he believed could stimulate thought in new ways. Deleuze often referred to artistic encounters as capable of generating new ways of thinking and relating. Jung appears to be no less positive when in the concluding part of his essay he calls upon the potentials in modern art, which, along with analytical psychology, might open thought beyond its containment in a claustrophobic and one-sided image.

The abstract idea of the State and the State-form

Jung used the term 'wholeness' frequently in his works. Often the term is accompanied by another, 'totality', referring to the total personality. He refers to the psyche as 'the totality of all psychic processes, conscious as well as unconscious' (1921: §797). The goal of wholeness is a distant one, Jung tells us, and by individuation he means 'the complete actualisation of the whole human being' (1934: §352). Elsewhere, Jung reminds us that individuation is 'the process by which a person

becomes a psychological "in-dividual", that is, a separate, indivis-
ible unity or "whole"' (1939: §490). In 'The undiscovered self' Jung
reflects on the 'fate of the individual human being' (1957: §497) in an
age of 'mass-mindedness' (ibid.: §§500, 511). At the end of the essay he
asks his readers to recognise an ethical imperative: that they recognise
the individual as 'that infinitesimal unit on whom a world depends'
(ibid.: §588). What has taken place such that Jung would be moved to
advocate for the necessity of such an 'individual'?

In his essay, Jung identifies a number of targets which he holds
as being responsible for the emergence of what he refers to as the
modern 'mass man' (ibid.: §§510, 511, 537, 538, 567). The targets
include the 'abstract idea of the State' (ibid.: §499), 'State-religion'[2]
(ibid.: §522) and a State-science whose methodology is predominately
'statistical' (ibid.: §§494, 495, 497, 499, 503, 507, 522, 523, 529; cf.
'statistical man', §537).[3] The problematic logical implications of the
abstract form of the State are closely bound up with a process of
'statistical levelling down' whose form Jung classifies as the 'rationalistic *Weltanschauung*' of the West (ibid.: §522; cf. §§523, 549, 553). The
logical implications of 'levelling down' involve processes of exclusion
which take as their object the 'irregular' (ibid.: §§494, 495). According
to Jung, the 'individual' is an exemplar of the 'irregular' and consequently a casualty of the exclusionary effects which levelling down
entails. He laments that 'it is not the universal and the regular that
characterise the individual, but rather the unique. He is not to be
understood as a recurrent unit but as something unique and singular' (ibid: §495). In this passage, Jung equates the terms 'universal',
'regular', and 'recurrent'. These terms serve the general function of
the 'rationalistic *Weltanschauung*', excluding the 'irregular', 'unique',
and 'singular'. The form of the *Weltanschauung* and of the 'abstract
idea of the State' is the same. Under this form, the organisation of
relations proceeds in accordance with certain assumptions and presuppositions; the assumption that man is a comparative unit results
in 'an abstract picture of man as an *average* unit from which all individual features have been removed' (ibid. par: 495; emphasis added).
Taken together, these processes of exclusion have an 'alienating effect'
(ibid.: §577) on the psyche of modern man.

In 1980 Deleuze and Guattari were also preoccupied with themes
similar to those that had engaged Jung some twenty years before. In

A Thousand Plateaus they generated a number of concepts that echo Jung's use of the concept 'mass' and the effects of 'levelling down', which he associated with the form of the 'rationalist *Weltanschuung*'. Chief among these concepts Deleuze and Guattari refer to the 'majority' and the 'majoritarian', which they present as 'the analytic fact of Nobody' (1980/1987: 105). By the term majoritarian they do not mean a greater relative quantity than something else, for example a minority.[4] Rather, 'majority implies a constant, of expression or content, serving as a standard measure by which to evaluate it' (ibid.). Deleuze and Guattari claim that '[m]ajority assumes a state of power and domination' (ibid.), and as an example of its representative man they refer to 'white, male, adult, "rational," etc., in short, the average European, the subject of enunciation' (ibid.: 292).[5] 'Majoritarian' man and 'mass man' refer to a 'Nobody': 'Majority is an abstract standard that can be said to include no one and thus speak in the name of nobody' (Conley 2005: 165). As we have seen, Jung takes account of something similar to the Nobody of this constant, standard and homogeneous majoritarian measure when he uses the term 'unit' to underscore the 'psychological effect of the statistical world-picture' (1957: §499).[6] As a 'recurrent', 'statistical', 'comparative', and 'average unit' (ibid.: §495), Jung's mass man is the product of a 'levelling down and a process of blurring that distorts the picture of reality into a conceptual average' (ibid.).

Both Jung and Deleuze–Guattari consider the formation of the mass and the majoritarian to have an intimate relationship with the State. Here a note of caution is required. When Jung refers to the 'abstract idea of the State' (1957: §499), he implies that he is not actively seeking to distinguish between specific States, historical or otherwise. In the essay Jung tends to single out totalitarian regimes because of their capacities for accelerating the production of mass-mindedness. He uses the term 'dictator States' (1957: §§510, 511, 514, 515, 517, 571, 580) when referring to totalitarian regimes and, as one might expect given the historical context of his essay (1957), there are references to Communism (ibid.: §§504, 515, 516, 523, 541, 544, 559, 568),[7] Russia, Stalin, China (ibid.: §517), and socialism (ibid.: §§511, 517).[8] But to conclude from this that Jung privileges some normative conception of the democratic State over other variations would be incorrect.[9] The State has a certain abstract form, and this form finds itself embodied in the rationalistic *Weltanschauung*. In their 'Treatise on nomadology', Deleuze and Guattari refer to the State-form directly:

> The State-form, as a form of interiority, has a tendency to reproduce itself, remaining identical to itself across its variations and easily recognizable within the limits of its poles, always seeking public recognition (there is no masked State). [...] Only thought is capable of inventing the fiction of a State that is universal by right, of elevating the State to the level of de jure universality [...]. If it is advantageous for thought to prop itself up with the State, it is no less advantageous for the State to extend itself in thought, and to be sanctioned by it as the unique, universal form. [...] The State gives thought a form of interiority, and thought gives that interiority a form of universality.
>
> (1980/1987: 360, 375, 376)

It is important to note that Deleuze and Guattari refer to the State-form as a form of interiority. In the 'Treatise', the system they are preoccupied with is the State or more broadly the political, but the form of interiority is not exclusive to the political. One can locate the form of interiority in other registers such as philosophical systems or other systems of thought. In the passage above, the authors indicate that the form of interiority can reproduce itself across variations. In 'The undiscovered self' the variations affected by the State-form include religion and science. In addition, Jung writes that for the mass man, 'the policy of the State is the supreme principle of thought and action. Indeed, this was the purpose for which he was enlightened, and accordingly the mass man grants the individual a right to exist *only in so far as he is a function of the State*' (1957: §510; emphasis added). Hence the State-form extends itself in thought accounting for the universality of presuppositions such as the recurrent and regular. When we try to distil the *form* of levelling down which Jung identifies with the rationalistic *Weltanschauung*, we should bear in mind Deleuze and Guattari's suggestion that the function of the State-form is 'capture'. Paul Patton summarises their account, reiterating that the 'essential function of the state is capture' but also that 'the underlying abstract form of the state is an interiority of some kind' (2000: 99). 'If it can help it', Deleuze and Guattari comment, 'the State does not dissociate itself from a process of capture of flows of all kinds, populations, commodities, money or capital, etc.' (1980/1987: 385–86). Levelling down captures relations by reducing them to the form of the same and interiorises them within a whole[10] or a milieu of interiority.

When religion 'compromises with the State', Jung says that he prefers 'to call it not "religion" but a "creed". A creed gives expression to a definite collective belief, whereas the word *religion* expresses a subjective relationship to certain metaphysical, extramundane factors' (ibid.: 507; emphasis in original).[11] Jung's criticism of religion as creed is echoed in Deleuze and Guattari's treatment of 'absolute religion' from the 'Treatise'. They claim that '[t]he absolute of religion is essentially a horizon that encompasses, and, if the absolute itself appears at a particular place, it does so in order to establish a solid and stable center for the global. [...] Religion is in this sense a piece in the State apparatus' (1980/1987: 382). When science compromises with the State, its form becomes statistical with its attendant implications such as levelling down. In the 'Treatise', Deleuze and Guattari label science 'Royal' or 'State-science' when it compromises with the State:

> Royal science is inseparable from a "hylomorphic" model implying both a form that organizes matter and a matter prepared for the form; it has often been shown that this schema derives less from technology or life than from a society divided into governors and governed, and later, intellectuals and manual laborers. What characterizes it is that all matter is assigned to content, while all form passes into expression.
>
> (1980/1987: 369)

If we read Jung's concerns about the extent to which thought, religion, and science compromise with the abstract idea of the State from a Deleuzian-Guattarian perspective, then the form of this compromise revolves around the form of interiority. This in turn concerns *relations* of interiority. In the previous passage, Deleuze and Guattari classify these relations as belonging to a schema that is hylomorphic, which involves the assumption of a 'transcendent, formal ordering of matter which generates two orders of being (form and content) that can only be related analogically' (Adkins 2015: 107). These two orders are ontologically discontinuous, and Deleuze and Guattari seek to account for an ontological continuum on which relations of interiority form one abstract pole (or tendency) but which includes relations of exteriority as another tendency. In the 'Treatise', the authors account for the difference between these two kinds of relations in the form of a reasonably straightforward metaphor. Referring to the difference between two board games, chess and Go, they write:

> Chess is a game of State, or of the court: the emperor of China played it. Chess pieces are coded; they have an internal nature and intrinsic properties from which their movements, situations, and confrontations derive. They have qualities; a knight remains a knight, a pawn a pawn, a bishop a bishop. Each is like a subject of the statement endowed with a relative power, and these relative powers combine in a subject of enunciation, that is, the chess player or the game's form of interiority. Go pieces, in contrast, are pellets, disks, simple arithmetic units, and have only an anonymous, collective, or third-person function: "It" makes a move. "It" could be a man, a woman, a louse, an elephant. Go pieces are elements of a nonsubjectified machine assemblage with no intrinsic properties, only situational ones. Thus the relations are very different in the two cases. [...] On the other hand, a Go piece has only a milieu of exteriority, or extrinsic relations with nebulas or constellations, according to which it fulfils functions of insertion or situation, such as bordering, encircling, shattering. [...] Finally, the space is not at all the same: in chess, it is a question of arranging a closed space for oneself, thus of going from one point to another, of occupying the maximum number of squares with the minimum number of pieces. In Go, it is a question of arraying oneself in an open space, of holding space, of maintaining the possibility of springing up at any point: the movement is not from one point to another, but becomes perpetual, without aim or destination, without departure or arrival. The "smooth" space of Go, as against the "striated" space of chess.
>
> (1980/1987: 352–53)

In this illustration, space is used to establish a context in which one can begin to approach the distinctions between relations of interiority (and its milieu) and relations of exteriority. We should recall that these distinctions are not intended as discontinuities but rather as tendencies on a continuum. Why is chess a game of State? Its space is already cut up (striated) and its pieces are coded according to their allowable moves and their shape. Although there are a vast number of permitted moves, the game is fundamentally static. Movement through striated space is highly controlled and the pieces have formalised identities that have been hierarchically organised in advance. Internal relations determine the function of the chessboard and pieces, and its milieu of interiority. Striated space is another term for a homogenous space of quantitative multiplicity in which relations are subordinate to a global dimensionality. As an abstract machine of capture, the State-form creates striated spaces which are homogenous and measurable and which constitute a milieu of interiority by drawing boundaries. These require common measures, which in turn enable a distribution of similarities and differences.

Jung does not employ spatial distinctions to articulate the differences between the rationalistic *Weltanschauung* and the role that the irregular might serve to resist its form. Instead he generates other concepts or uses existing ones in a very novel way. As we have seen, he sets up a distinction between the individual and the mass man. Likewise, he draws the reader's attention to the notion of the 'whole man' (1957: §§523, 553, 561). These are concepts of resistance or 'war-machines'[12] (to adopt another concept from Deleuze and Guattari's 'Treatise'). Jung characterises the whole man as an irrational datum, 'the *concrete* man as opposed to the unreal ideal or "normal" man' (ibid.: §498; emphasis in original). What are the capabilities of the whole man? What can he/she do? This is an ethical question in the Spinozistic sense of ethics as an expansion of what a body can do. The whole man is capable of relating in ways that are not captured or excluded by the State-form. Adkins comments that '[i]t is precisely for this reason that the war machine is always trying to ward off the state. [...] The state converts the war machine's exteriority to a self-same interiority' (2015: 113). These modes of relating are experimental, that is, their effects cannot be fully determined in advance; but this does not mean that no influence is exerted on others or the world.

In the 'Treatise', Deleuze and Guattari introduce a number of concepts which are used for thinking through the implications of ways of relating which are exterior to, or outside, those of the State-form. Most of the time they refer to the nomad, nomadic, and nomadicism,[13] situating these in relation to different contexts (e.g. space, language, art, thought, and so on). Elsewhere in *A Thousand Plateaus* they refer to processes such as 'becoming-revolutionary' (1980/1987: 292) and 'becoming-minoritarian' (ibid.: 106–7). They declare that '[t]here is no becoming-majoritarian; majority is never a becoming' (ibid.: 107), meaning that in becoming-minoritarian one does not aim at acquiring a new majority and a new constant. Rather, the figure of a minoritarian consciousness, Deleuze and Guattari assert:

> continually oversteps the representative threshold of the majoritarian standard, by excess or default. In erecting the figure of a universal minoritarian consciousness, one addresses powers (*puissances*) of becoming that belong to a different realm from that of Power (*Pouvoir*) and Domination. Continuous variation constitutes the becoming-minoritarian of everybody, as opposed to the majoritarian Fact of Nobody.
>
> (1980/1987: 106)

Are we entitled to equate this universal figure of minoritarian consciousness with the figure of the whole man and the individual presented in 'The undiscovered self'? As a continuous variation, the becoming peculiar to minoritarian consciousness is a kind of metamorphosis, a potential to deviate from the standard or unit that defines the mass and the majority. Resistance to the abstract idea of the State is developed in the minoritarian consciousness of the whole man who is capable of experimenting with relations engendering heterogeneous connections which are open to the outside. Finally, we might recall some of Jung's earliest sentiments from his final lecture to the *Zofingiaverein* from 1899:[14] '[t]o be sure, the normal man is not a quantity acknowledged by public statute, but rather is the product of tacit convention, a thing that exists everywhere and nowhere' (1899: §246). The image of the whole man that Jung presents us with over fifty years later in 'The undiscovered self' calls to this image of the normal man which, as a man of nowhere, is an analytic fact of Nobody and whose everywhere is majoritarian, in contrast to the becoming-minoritarian of everybody.

Jung's critique of the 'image of thought' and its 'orientation' in 'The undiscovered self'

In the previous section, I identified a number of conceptual affinities between Jung's essay 'The undiscovered self' and Deleuze/Guattari's 'Treatise on nomadology' from *A Thousand Plateaus*. We saw that these writers were equally concerned with the logical and ethical implications of the exclusory effects that they considered certain forms of relations could engender in thought and society. In what follows I want to return to Jung's essay and examine the ways in which he accounts for the genesis of the habits of thought peculiar to the mass man and what he tells us about resisting these habits. Likewise, I will return to the work of Deleuze and of Deleuze and Guattari in order to assist this examination. In this section, my focus is primarily on the system of thought rather than the State-form. What remains common to both systems is the form of interiority.

In his essay, Jung offers the following erudite synopsis of the genesis of the alienating effects of exclusion on the psyche of modern man:

> His consciousness therefore *orientates* itself chiefly by observing and investigating the world around him, and it is to the latter's peculiarities that he must adapt his psychic and technical resources. This task is so exacting, and its fulfilment so profitable, that he forgets himself in the process, losing sight of his instinctual nature and *putting his own conception of himself in place of his real being*. In this way he slips imperceptibly into a purely *conceptual world* where the products of his conscious activity progressively take the place of reality.
>
> (Jung 1957: §557; emphasis added)

Jung refers to a certain orientation of thought towards the conceptual which gradually engenders an image of thought that becomes exacting, that is, fixed. Man puts his own image or conception of himself in the place of other images; in other words, man takes 'one image as the source and ground of all other images, without accounting for how this image of all imaging is possible' (Colebrook 2010: 184–85). This is exactly what Jung laments when in 1937 he accounts for the death of God as a process whereby God's image dissolves into the common man. The common man (like the mass man) 'suffers from a hubris of consciousness that borders on the pathological'. Jung avers that '[t]his psychic condition in the individual corresponds by and large to the hypertrophy and totalitarian pretentions of the idealised State' (1938/ 1940: §141). The death of God (first heralded by Friedrich Nietzsche [1844–1900]) was the death of an image of God that had become too closely grounded in our own common image. '[W]ith Nietzsche', Jung says ' "God is dead." Yet it would be truer to say, "He has put off *our image*, and where shall we find him again?" ' (ibid.: 144; emphasis added). What is lost in this process is an understanding of the genesis of 'our image' and how it came to be so dominant and all-pervasive.

One of the less explicit preoccupations of Jung's essay concerns a mass projection with a one-sided orientation and image of thought. This collective projection is facilitated by the State apparatus when it is universalised in the discourse of creeds and the methodologies of statistical science. The collective identification with this image is marked by Jung as 'the triumph of the Goddess of Reason' and he says that it testifies to 'a general neuroticizing of modern man' (1957: §553). Elsewhere in the essay, Jung argues that the 'supremacy' and 'worship of the word' (*logos*) 'was necessary at a certain phase of man's development' (ibid.: §554). This sentiment is also echoed in the following: '[o]nly when conditions have altered so drastically that there is an unendurable rift between the outer situation and our ideas, now become antiquated, does the general problem of our *Weltanschauung* or philosophy of life, arise' (1957: §549). In these passages one can discern an emphasis on a necessary or inevitable diremption of modern man, which results in collective neurosis. In her critical study of the recent ascendency of the image of the organism in 'contemporary modern vitalisms',[15] Claire Colebrook (a Deleuzian scholar) claims that 'it is the diremption of modern man – and all the false problems, neuroses, alienations and illusions that he brings in train – that allows this non-organic, abstract, ideal, spiritual or properly machinic and differential life to be intuited' (2010: 177). This follows in the train of 'necessary illusions [...] leading the way to an intuition of life as essentially productive of its own misrecognition' (ibid.). A collective projection and identification with a one-sided image may be a consequence of 'the organism's tendency to territorialise or re-territorialise all relations around the image of its own illusory unity' (ibid.: 143).

Jung's comment that alienated modern man 'slips imperceptibly into a purely conceptual world' (1957: §557) gestures to his awareness of the counter-efficient, neurotic effects of this process of universalisation, capture, and territorialisation. I include these points to show that scrutiny of collective projection is a critical act, one that is only possible 'after trauma – after the self has experienced what is other than itself as an alien infraction' (Colebrook 2010: 176). On a collective level this testifies to those moments of 'extreme isolation, impoverishment and detachment from "life" that man recognises as a power to create distorting, truncated, illogical and sterile images' (ibid.: 180).

Orientation to an image of thought is another way of expressing a certain way of *relating* to an image. I postulate that in 'The undiscovered self' Jung is proposing an ethical re-orientation of the way we relate to each other and the world via a new image. This image is closely aligned with the way he presents the positive concept of the individual and the whole man in the essay. As we shall see, the whole man acts as a kind of conceptual persona for Jung in his essay. I borrow 'conceptual personae' from the last work by Deleuze and Guattari, *What is Philosophy?* (1991/1994). They write that 'philosophy is the art of forming, inventing, and fabricating concepts' and that 'concepts need conceptual personae that play a part in their definition' (ibid.: 2). The concept is a 'presence that is intrinsic to thought, a condition of possibility of thought itself, a living category, a transcendental lived reality' (ibid.: 3). 'Concepts are not waiting for us ready-made, like heavenly bodies. There is no heaven for concepts. They must be invented, fabricated, or rather created and would be nothing without their creator's signature' (ibid.: 5).

Jung's presentation of the concepts 'whole man' and 'individual' in the essay can be regarded as transformative concepts. Although the term 'individual' is very common and often carries with it certain implicit presuppositions, Jung's critical use of the term in the essay is novel and challenging. In those passages from 'The undiscovered self' where Jung criticises mass and collective opinion (e.g. 1957: §§503, 535, 554), he comes close to Deleuze's criticism of the image of thought (which forms the basis of Deleuze's third chapter of *Difference and Repetition*). In this criticism Deleuze takes Descartes' famous 'I think therefore I am' to task for presupposing too much, namely 'what it means to be and to think [...] and that no one can deny that to doubt is to think, and to think is to be. [...] *Everybody knows, no one can deny*, is the form of representation and the discourse of the representative' (1968/1994: 130; emphasis in original). According to Deleuze, the *doxa* of common-sense and good-sense forms the implicit presupposition of philosophy as *cogitatio natura universalis*, and he suggests that we 'may call this image of thought a dogmatic, orthodox or moral image' (ibid.: 131). What is it that can challenge this image of thought? I suggest that Jung's deployment of the individual and the whole man might have something in common with the way in which Deleuze and Guattari present the 'Idiot' as a conceptual persona capable of resisting this image (1991/1994: 62). In *Difference and Repetition*, Deleuze comments:

> At the risk of playing the idiot, do so in the Russian manner: that of an underground man who recognises himself no more in the subjective presuppositions of a natural capacity for thought than in the objective presuppositions of a culture of the times, and lacks the compass with which to make a circle. Such a one is the Untimely, neither temporal nor eternal.
>
> (1968/1994: 130)

We ask if Jung's notion of the individual and whole man might also have affinities with the underground man, one with the 'necessary modesty':

> not managing to know what everybody knows, and modestly denying what everybody is supposed to recognise. Someone who neither allows himself to be represented nor wishes to represent anything. Not an individual endowed with good will and a natural capacity for thought, but an individual full of ill will who does not manage to think, either naturally or conceptually.
>
> (1968/1994: 130)

When Jung criticises the rationalist *Weltanschauung* and proposes an alternative to 'the triumph of the Goddess of Reason' (1957: §553), it is reason itself that is subjected to critique, given the way it has become orientated by the established values of the abstract idea of the State. We have seen how these values serve to exclude, how they become lodged in an image of thought which sustains collective opinion in a one-sided manner: '[t]he image of thought is the only figure in which *doxa* is universalised by being elevated to the rational level' (Deleuze 1968/ 1994: 134). If we read Jung's essay with these comments in mind, then he can be regarded as an 'untimely', 'private thinker',[16] a voice among other 'isolated and passionate cries' which are isolated on account of the fact that 'they deny what everybody knows [...]. And passionate, since they deny that which, it is said, nobody can deny' (ibid.: 130). In the words of Bruce Baugh: 'The private thinker is unreasonable because Reason is nothing but the guarantor of the ideas of "everyone", and the private thinker is incapable of going along with the crowd, even at the cost of being misunderstood and despised' (2015: 315).

Becoming estranged

Returning to the passage from 'The undiscovered self' that I drew from earlier (1957: §557), it is noteworthy that Jung refers to the real being of man and his instinctual foundations as having become uprooted. Such terms might imply a kind of original[17] image or a natural way of relating before the fall of modernity.[18] But such an assessment would be too simplistic. Elsewhere in the essay Jung calls on a positive power of 'estrangement' (1957: §§507, 557) that can be contrasted with the alienating and exclusionary effects propagated by the prevailing image of thought. During encounters with the 'extramundane' (ibid.: pars, 507, 508, 509, 511, 514, 543),[19] an estranging *distancing* from the image of thought occurs. At times Jung refers to this estrangement as involving an 'immediate inner experience' (1957: §592) or an 'immediate relation with God' (ibid.: §§563, 564).[20] In becoming estranged from a prevailing normative image, potentials for imaging (which were formerly excluded by this image, or captured by it and reduced to the form of the same) are freed. This may be characterised as a positive process of disembodiment in the sense that a normative image of thought (for example, what Jung calls the statistical man or the mass man) is an image from which one is becoming estranged. Nonetheless, a normative image of the self is a rather vague characterisation. Colebrook offers some articulation in the following context:

> The normative image of the artwork is tied closely to the normative image of the self, and both are premised on a norm of organic

life: the proper self is a well-formed whole in which there is not an imposed or centered form so much as a dynamic interaction of constantly re-engaged parts, all contributing to the ongoing coherence of a well-bounded unity.

(2010: 69)

Colebrook is decidedly critical of this image of the bounded 'whole', a whole which is often assumed to be maintained and regulated via a fixed inventory of transcendental conditions or sensory-motor habits. Other Deleuzian scholars such as Rosi Braidotti do not refer to a normative image directly, but critically consider normative features of the modern liberal subject such as the common-sense notion that only stable identities reposing on firms grounds of rational and moral universalism can ensure ethical probity, moral and political agency, and basic human decency (2012: 170). A normative image of the liberal individual with a universalistic or individual core (moral intentionality/rational consciousness) is not presupposed by Jung as a necessary condition for ethics; in its place a non-unitary, relational vision of the subject as whole is accorded priority. To this extent, Jung has something in common with post-structuralist philosophies in that he promotes the 'dissolution of the hard-core self of liberal individualism' (Braidotti 2012: 186) and tacitly advocates an 'ethics of depersonalisation', achieving a 'post-identity or non-unitary vision of the self' which requires 'the dis-identification from established references' (ibid.). Estrangement from an organic image of the whole is disembodying in the sense that the organisation of its internal relations is freed from subordination to a pre-given whole. Relations that were not considered proper to the milieu in which the organic image had been situated are opened up onto an outside.[21] Being orientated by an image of thought that is too closely grounded in the conditioned (or too much like an organic whole) presupposes a certain distribution of relations that can have negative logical and ethical implications. These implications can be registered at different levels: at the level of the abstract idea of the State (Jung's preoccupation in 'The undiscovered self'), at the level of thought (Deleuze's preoccupation in *Difference and Repetition*), and at the level of life (or the organism, which is one register among others that preoccupy Deleuze and Guattari in *A Thousand Plateaus*).[22]

The reciprocity between this image and the State engenders a one-sidedness which can reach epidemic (mass) proportions. The organisation and distribution of relations is channelled through thought and through institutions such as religion and science. In disorganising this image, the relation *to* the image of thought alters significantly:

> It would not, therefore, be a question of evaluating images, theories or art works on the basis of their proximity to the lived; it would not be a question of judging images according to their attainability or similarity to what is recognised or recognisable. What needs to be rethought is not the nature and content of images [...] but the *relation to images*.
>
> (Colebrook 2010: 115–16; emphasis in original)

What is important in this passage is the emphasis on non-organic images or those which are estranged to the point of bearing no relation with the recognised of common opinion. Considered in this way, Jung's reflection on the process of estrangement can be read as a commentary on ways of re-organising relations which are opened up during encounters with the extramundane, as he calls it. The individual or whole man can engage potentials in new ways that were formerly prohibited.

One of the reasons for the numerous references to art and artists (untimely and private thinkers) in the work of Deleuze and Deleuze/Guattari[23] relates to their interest in the estranging and transformative effects that ideas and artistic works can evoke in the encounter. They attempt to ally these effects with concepts, accounting for a philosophical process of concept creation. In relation to this it might be worth recalling the following point on which Deleuze insisted:

> Something in the world forces us to think. This something is an object not of recognition but of a fundamental *encounter*. What is encountered may be Socrates, a temple or a demon. It may be grasped in a range of affective tones: wonder, love, hatred, suffering. In whichever tone, its primary characteristic is that it can only be sensed.
>
> (1968/1994: 139; emphasis original)

Art and extramundane encounters

Jung tends to territorialise estranging encounters with the extramundane on to the more traditional language of theology, but we need to recall that he takes theology to task when 'it compromises with the State' and 'compromises with mundane reality' (1957: §507). Furthermore, at the end of 'The undiscovered self', Jung suggests the possibility of an alliance between his analytical psychology and what he calls modern art. He recognises that this art-form has 'turned away from the old object-relationship toward the dark chaos' (ibid.: §584) and that it has opened up relations in such a way that they are no longer dependent on recognition. Jung claims that modern art is an 'excellent example: though seeming to deal with aesthetic problems, it is really performing a work of psychological education on the public by breaking down and destroying their previous aesthetic views of what is beautiful in form and meaningful in content' (ibid.). In other words, it breaks down an image of thought. Nevertheless, Jung remains ambivalent about this 'education', adding that 'art, so far as we can judge it, has not yet discovered in this darkness what it is that could hold all men together and give expression to their psychic wholeness' (ibid.). In spite of this, he concludes that 'since reflection seems to be needed for this purpose, it may be that such discoveries are reserved for other fields of endeavour' (ibid.). Potential alliances between different fields of endeavour are something that Jung is open to.[24]

Deleuze and Guattari's philosophy has been characterised as one that actively forms (machinic) alliances with non-philosophies, such as art, cinema, and science. In these alliances philosophy does not claim any right to judge or assume any position of superiority (Deleuze 1968/1994: xvi; Lambert 2003: 18–19). This strategy is employed by Deleuze and by Deleuze and Guattari in their philosophy at large. Extramundane encounters in their work are most often drawn from aesthetic examples and from the world of ideas, past and present. It is arguably for this reason that Jung's work found its way directly into the hands of Deleuze and encouraged him to write his 1961 essay 'From Sacher-Masoch to masochism', in which 'we find Deleuze entranced by Jung's labyrinthine 1912 book *Transformations and Symbols of the Libido*' (Kerslake 2004: 135).[25] In his work, Jung established alliances with what we might call non-psychologies; for instance, in his collaboration with Wolfgang Pauli (1900–1958) an alliance was formed with quantum physics. Jung's more orthodox sources of alliance included mythology, religion, and certain branches of philosophy. Indeed, alliance formation appears to be at the heart of his empiricism.[26] In combination, these varied sources form a 'machinic assemblage'; in other words, analytical psychology does not and cannot work all by itself: it needs 'other machines that fit into its apparatus or assemblage and provide it with contents in order to work, in order to produce concepts' (Lambert 2012: 19).

Is it noteworthy that Jung includes comment on modern art in the closing passages of 'The undiscovered self' as if art, with analytical psychology, had a role to play in an alliance of resistance against the alienating orientation of the image of thought? There are a number of reasons why it might be. Firstly, it has already been established that Jung finds something of value in the power of modern art to destabilise object-recognition. From a Deleuzian perspective, this can be read as gesturing to ways of relating to images which do not presuppose a certain exclusionary distribution and organisation of relations. Secondly, Jung's inclusion of modern art in his essay also points to another domain in which the extramundane can be encountered. An encounter with God, an encounter with the unconscious, and encounters with modern art reinforce a theme that runs throughout Jung's essay, i.e. the destabilisation of the distinction between the inner and the outer.[27] Roderick Main makes a related point:

> Although the collective unconscious is not structured socially, its field of influence inescapably includes society; and although the individuating person's obligations are not imposed directly from the outer, social order, they emerge inwardly partly as a response to and in a form that encompasses the outer, social and indeed environmental order.
>
> (2004: 142)

Jung tends to classify extramundane encounters as examples of immediate inner experience (1957: §592). What is the status of inner when it is thought of in terms of relations? The inner is not a private and personal location. It is not the 'possession of a subjective interiority or thought' (Adkins 2015: 117). Rather, the form of the inner is an exteriority. In the context of 'The undiscovered self', which deals with the negative effects of an orientation to an image of thought whose form is embodied in the abstract idea of the State, the outer corresponds to a form of interiority with respect to the organisation of its relations. Employing some of Main's terms above, the outer order cannot be the cause of obligations because the form by which it organises relations is diametrically at odds with the form of exteriority that obligates the whole man and the private thinker. Modern art, which problematises the inner/outer binary in terms of exteriority/interiority relations and which in Jung's view performs a 'work of psychological education on the public' (1957: §584), is capable of presenting images which break with the organic form of representation and recognition that characterises object-recognition and the orientation of the 'conceptual world' (ibid.: §557). It can encompass the outer, social, and environmental because in breaking with old images, new ways and modes of relating may be revealed which open experimental pathways with 'this world' or worlds that had formerly been obscured or excluded. To engage with this world, according to Deleuze, necessitates a belief, but one that is 'no longer addressed to a different or transformed world':

> Man is in the world as if in a pure optical and sound situation. The reaction of which man has been dispossessed can be replaced only by belief. Only belief in the world can reconnect man to what he sees and hears. [...] Restoring our belief in the world – this is the power of modern cinema (when it stops being bad). [...] What is certain is that believing is no longer believing in another world, or in a transformed world. It is only, it is simply believing in the body.
> (1989: 172)[28]

For Deleuze, an inward response to the outer orientation of the mass man would involve a belief in this world. In his 'Concerning the archetypes, with special reference to the anima concept' (1936/1954), Jung wrote that the anima (soul or psyche) was inseparable from the world: 'Its nature [the psyche] shows itself not merely in the personal sphere, or in the instinctual or social, but in phenomena of worldwide distribution. So if we want to understand the psyche, we have to include the whole world' (ibid.: §114).[29] Elsewhere Jung claimed that '[i]ndividuation does not shut one out from the world, but gathers the world to oneself' (1947/1954: §432).[30] What opens this world up are estranging encounters and, as we have seen, Jung has referred to these as 'extramundane', including art as a venue for their engagement. For Deleuze and Deleuze/Guattari these encounters can take place across numerous different registers and their philosophy is in part a study of estranging images, a practice they sometimes refer to as noology. In the 'Treatise' they offer this definition:

> Noology, which is distinct from ideology, is precisely the study of images of thought, and their historicity. [...] noology is confronted by counterthoughts, which are violent in their acts and discontinuous in their appearance, and whose existence is mobile in history. These are acts of a "private thinker", as opposed to the public professor: Kierkegaard, Nietzsche, or even Shestov. Wherever they dwell, it is the steppe or the desert. They destroy images.
>
> (1980/1987: 376)

'The undiscovered self' with its innovative use of concepts such as the mass man might be read as a study of images. In this way Jung can be called a private thinker and his essay embodies an inward response that encompasses this world. In the 'Treatise', Deleuze and Guattari refer to the private thinker as experiencing a certain kind of solitude. They qualify their use of the term private thinker, stating that this 'is not a satisfactory expression, because it exaggerates interiority, when it is a question of *outside thought*. [...] And this form of exteriority of thought is not at all symmetrical to the form of interiority' (1980/1987: 376, 377).[31] They give further reasons for this qualification. Firstly, 'to place thought in an immediate relation with the outside, with the forces of the outside, in short to make thought a war machine, is a strange undertaking'. Secondly, they say that '[a]lthough it is true that this counterthought attests to an absolute solitude, it is an extremely populous solitude like the desert itself, a solitude already intertwined with a people to come, one that invokes and awaits that people, existing only through it, though it is not yet here' (ibid.: 376–77). Thinking of the inner that Jung refers to so often in 'The undiscovered self' as a populous solitude might serve to de-emphasise an epistemological and ontological discontinuity that can become entrenched in the inner/

outer distinction. Jung's use of the concept of mass as well as his novel use of the terms 'individual' and 'whole man' can be read as opening up an outside thought by exposing the conditions and genesis of what organises relations in an exclusory fashion (the abstract idea of the State) and at the same time advocating for an engagement with the extramundane across different registers. Like Deleuze and Guattari's 'Treatise', Jung's essay has an untimely quality.

Concluding remarks

The potential influence of Jung's essay, its public or educational role cannot be determined in advance. It is not the work of a public professor or what Deleuze and Guattari also call a 'State-thinker' or 'man of the State' (1980/1987: 25, 268, 269, 356, 378, 482) because it does not compromise with the 'State-form' (ibid.: 376). Indeed, Jung's essay critically exposes the logical and ethical implications of relations when thought, the church, and science compromise with the State-form. The outcomes of the essay are experimental and the work is in solidarity with 'a new earth and people that do not yet exist', an 'oppressed, bastard, lower, anarchical and irretrievably minor race', as Deleuze and Guattari put it (1991/1994: 108–9).[32] The *uses* that concepts are put to by Jung in the essay should not be read as harbouring any pretensions to the erection of a new normativity, majority, or mass of the future.[33] Rather, their use gestures to the potential creation of pockets of resistance, whose form is experimental. Wholeness in this context is an ethical experimental practice or performance with relations that 'liberate life and thought from already constituted relations and extended quantities but not by appealing to some pure life before all differentiation' (Colebrook 2010: 151). Deleuze and Guattari's philosophical method is often guided by the question: 'what would thinking be if it were detached from the organised body of self-constituting man and placed in relation to other differentials? [...] becoming-imperceptible, or the thought of *not* being, not maintaining oneself, experimenting not with annihilation and return to anti-self-consciousness' but with 'approximation to zero' (ibid.: 151, 152).

In 'The undiscovered self', Jung raises awareness of the period of extreme isolation that man is undergoing. From a Deleuzian perspective, this is not to be understood as isolation from a natural way of relating; rather, it testifies to a *power* to create images and experimental ways of relating to them. To become *critically* and *creatively* aware of this power involves estranging encounters and for Deleuze and Guattari these can be used to generate concepts which resist the hegemonic effects that the prevailing one-sided image tends to exert on relations.

Acknowledgement

Work on this chapter was supported by the Arts and Humanities Research Council [AH/N003853/1].

Notes

1 Throughout this chapter the word 'State' is given an initial capital, as in the English translations of both Jung's 'The undiscovered self' (1957) and Deleuze and Guattari's 'Treatise on nomadology' in *A Thousand Plateaus* (1980/1987: 409–92).

2 Or more generally religion governed by 'creeds' (Jung 1957: §507; see below).

3 Roderick Main (following Peter Homans) claims that 'Jung's understanding of modern society was "identical to that of the theory of mass society" – a theory which, along with Marxism, is "the most prevalent and widely known theory of modernity". The modern form of this theory originated in the work of Max Scheler, José Ortega, and Karl Mannheim' (2004: 136; Homans 1995: 178, 174).

4 The statistical number of minorities may in actuality be greater than that of the majority: 'A minority can be numerous, or even infinite; so can a majority. What distinguishes them is that in the case of a majority the relation internal to the number constitutes a set that may be finite or infinite, but is always denumerable, whereas the minority is defined as a nondenumerable set, however many elements it may have' (Deleuze and Guattari 1987: 469–70). Deleuze and Guattari also claim that 'the use of the number as a numeral, as a statistical element, is proper to the numbered number of the State, not to the numbering number' (1980/ 1987: 390). One might also compare this to Jung's critical comments on 'large numbers' from his essay (1957: §§503, 524, 535, 538, 539). It is clear from the essay that Jung tends to associate the 'mass' with large numbers.

5 We might compare this with Jung's acknowledgement that 'the European has also to answer for all the crimes he has committed against the coloured races during the process of colonization. In this respect the white man carries a very heavy burden indeed. It shows a picture of the common human shadow that could hardly be painted in blacker colours' (1957: §571; cf. Deleuze and Guattari's critical comments on the 'Face' of Christ as 'white' and what they call the 'white wall/black hole system' [1980/1987: 167–88]).

6 Jung's concerns about 'statistical' science are evident from his earliest lectures, the *Zofingia Lectures* (1896–1899). 'To be sure, the normal man is not a quantity acknowledged by public statute, but rather is the product of tacit convention, a thing that exists everywhere and *nowhere* [...] Just as a Paris cellar now harbours a *standard meter* by which all other instruments of measurement are calibrated, so, in an indetectable place inside the heads of scientific-minded men, there exists the standard of the normal man that is used to calibrate all scientific-philosophical traits' (1983: §246; emphasis added; cf.: §287. See Bishop 1995: 42).

7 Jung differentiates between historical variations, e.g. 'primitive communism' (1957: §503) and Marxism (ibid.: §§522, 523, 549, 568).

8 Cf. Main 2004: 117–21, 135–38.

9 Deleuze and Guattari assert that the State is an 'abstract machine of overcoding' (1980/1987: 230), with a specific form and a function before any concrete historical incarnation.

10 A recurring theme throughout all of Deleuze's thought, including with Guattari, concerns relations of the 'whole' (*tout*). Deleuze's persistent criticisms of a 'logical', 'organic unity'/'organic totality' and internal relations are situated across many different registers throughout his works (history, literature, art, cinema, politics, biology), and the notion of the 'whole' frequently appears with them. Many Deleuzians are critical of the term 'holism' (e.g. DeLanda 2009: 37) because they tend to equate this with organicism (e.g. Colebrook 2010: 141–45) and with the relations of interiority that Deleuze tends to identify with organic unity/totality (e.g. Deleuze 1966/2000: 113–16, 161, 163; 1983/1986: 95–96, 322–23, 326–27; cf. 'closed' and 'open' whole/s [1983/1986: 9–11, 16–20; Deleuze and Guattari 1991/1994: 105]).

11 Under these circumstances of 'compromise', Jung asserts that '[t]he State takes the place of God' and that if '[t]he policy of the State is exalted to a creed, the leader or party boss becomes a demigod beyond good and evil' (1957: §511).

12 It should be noted that the object of the 'war machine' is not war in the conventional sense but the conditions of creative mutation and change (see Patton 2000: 109–10; cf. Deleuze and Guattari 1980/1987: 229–30).

13 Also nomad science, nomad space, nomad war-machine, nomad art, nomad thought (see Deleuze and Guattari 1980/1987: 359–423).

14 Jung delivered these lectures as a student in the years 1896–1899 between the ages of twenty-one and twenty-three. In May 1895 he became a member of the *Zofingiaverein*, a Swiss Student Fraternity, and was elected Chairperson of the Basle section during the winter term of 1897/98.

15 E.g. Humberto Maturana and Francisco Varela's model of living systems, Andy Clark's anti-Cartesian positing of an extended mind, and the Gaia hypothesis. These are targeted in Colebrook's study.

16 In the 'Treatise', Deleuze and Guattari refer to the 'private thinker' in a manner reminiscent of their treatment of the conceptual persona of the 'Idiot' (1980/1987: 376). Their selection and presentation of certain 'private thinkers' and modern artists as case studies dispenses with any excavation of their personal past in a manner reminiscent of Jung's distinction between 'visionary art' and 'psychological art' (1930/1950: §139).

17 For example, he refers to building a 'bridge to the original man' as a solution to the alienating effects of the rationalist *Weltanschauung* (1957: §549).

18 As Colebrook notes: 'perhaps the most dominant form of this narrative, and one that has a great deal of force at present, is the lapse into Cartesianism: current diagnoses of the state of play in philosophy, neuroscience, and everyday thinking lament the ways in which, following Descartes' error we mistake the mind for a distinct substance, and then imagine knowledge as some mode of picturing or information processing' (2010: 130).

19 In the *Zofingia Lectures* Jung uses the term 'supermundane' in a similar way (1983: §287). Jane Bennett surveys the narratives of 'loss' that inform many disenchantment 'tales' (2001: 56–90). Bennett refers to a 'Deleuzean [*sic*] kind of enchantment, where wonders persist in a rhizomatic world without intrinsic purpose or divinity, or the "subjective necessity" (again Kant's phrase) of assuming telos or God' (ibid.: 34).

20 These notions of 'immediate' experience appear in Jung's earliest lectures (1896–1899) where he refers to the idea of a *unio mystica* (1983: §§225, 257, 259, 265, 272, 289, 290). He contrasts this with the 'ominous taint of Kantian subjectivism' (ibid.: §251; cf. Paul Bishop, 1995: 42) that he identifies in the theology of Albrecht Ritschl (1822–1899). By 'Kantian subjectivism' I think Jung had in mind Kant's philosophical commitment to a 'rational faith' (*Vernunftglaube*), which Kant espoused in part as response to the pantheism controversy, opposing with some vehemence Friedrich Heinrich Jacobi's (1743–1819) *salto mortale* (a leap of faith).

21 Disembodiment is often thought of as something negative because of its association with Cartesianism and attendant disenchantment narratives. However, Colebrook comments that Deleuze and Guattari's thought is sometimes preoccupied by a 'perverse Cartesianism... that does not react against Descartes because he dehumanised life by rendering man into a ghostly disembodied subject, but because *res cogitans* was too much like a living body' (2010: 144).

22 E.g. '[N]ot all Life is confined to the organic strata: rather, the organism is that which life sets against itself in order to limit itself, and there is a life all the more intense, all the more powerful for being anorganic. There are also nonhuman Becomings of human beings that overspill the anthropomorphic strata in all directions' (1980/1987: 503).

23 E.g. *Proust and Signs* (1966/2000); *Francis Bacon: The Logic of Sensation* (1981/2003); *Cinema I* (1983/1986) and *Cinema II* (1985/1989), and in collaboration with Guattari, e.g. *Kafka: Toward a Minor Literature* (1986).

24 For example, in 1945 Jung writes: 'Science *qua* science has no boundaries, and there is no speciality whatever that can boast of complete self-sufficiency. Any speciality is bound to spill over its borders and to encroach on adjoining territory if it is to lay serious claim to the status of a science' (1945: §212)

25 Kerslake writes that 'Deleuze's central thesis is that masochism must be conceived as a *perverse realisation of the fantasy of incest* – on condition that incest is taken in its "more profound" significance as a symbol of rebirth, as Jung claims' (2004: 135). Positive references to Jung's work appear in Deleuze's *Difference and Repetition* where Deleuze rhetorically asks: Was not one of the most important points of Jung's theory already to be found here: the force of 'questioning' in the unconscious, the conception of the unconscious as an unconscious of 'problems' and 'tasks'? Drawing out the consequences of this led Jung to the discovery of a process of differentiation more profound than the resulting oppositions (see *The Ego and the Unconscious*)' (1994: 317, n. 17). This remark forms the basis of Kerslake's detailed study of the relationship between Bergson, Kant, Jung and Deleuze (2007).

26 Sean McGrath alludes to this when he claims that the 'empirical component to analytical psychology' is 'abductive, not inductive': 'The explanatory account itself is not deduced from the empirical facts: its sources are varied: the history of mythology, religion, and philosophy, as well as Jung's own not infrequent flights of *a priori* speculation. Abduction "leads away" (*ab-ducere*) from the empirical facts to be explained and constructs, on the basis of logical, imaginative, and intuitive moves, a speculative account of how those facts could be possible' (2014: 30).

27 Jung appears to de-emphasise the 'outer world' (e.g. 1957: §§507, 549), the 'external' (ibid.: §§508, 511, 529, 561, 563), and the 'worldly' (ibid.: §§514, 543, 563, 567) in the essay and valorise the 'inner' (ibid.: §§511, 516, 519, 521, 529, 533, 537, 542, 561). A potential consequence of this emphasis on the 'inner' is to locate 'psychological reality and the nature of the self more within the private sector' (Homans 1995: 142–43), the process of individuation being 'entirely psychical not social' with an endpoint that 'is a pure and intensely privatised self, liberated from all obligation imposed from without by the social order' (ibid.: 143).

28 Cf.: '[I]t may be that living in this world, in this life, becomes our most difficult task, or the task of a mode of existence still to be discovered or our plane of immanence today' (Deleuze and Guattari 1991/1994:75).

29 Cf. Bishop 2009: 154.

30 Cf. Main 2004: 140. On this sentence Bishop comments that 'in the definition of 'individuation'… given in that work, Jung makes the famous remark *Individuation schließt die Welt nicht aus, sondern ein*, inaccurately but wonderfully translated by R.F.C. Hull as "individuation does not shut one out from the world, but gathers the world to oneself"' (2008: 161). Bishop's translation is: 'individuation does not exclude, but includes, the world'.

31 See Michel Foucault's analysis of Maurice Blanchot and the form of exteriority of thought: 'La pensée du dehors' ,*Critique*, no. 229 (June 1966): 523–48.

32 Jung appears to call on such a people when he declares that the 'spiritual transformation of mankind… may not set in for hundreds of years' (1957: §583).

33 Nevertheless, Jung also states that he would like to see the 'effect on *all* individuals' (1957: §583). Would this be to erect another 'majority' or 'consensus' of the future?

References

Adkins, B. (2015). What is a literature of war?: Kleist, Kant and nomadology. In C. Lundy and D. Voss (Eds.), *At the Edges of Thought: Deleuze and Post-Kantian Philosophy*, 105–22. Edinburgh: Edinburgh University Press.

Baugh, B. (2015). Private thinkers, untimely thoughts: Deleuze, Shestov and Fondane. *Continental Philosophy Review* 48(3): 313–39.

Bennett, J. (2001). *The Enchantment of Modern Life: Attachments, Crossings, and Ethics*. Princeton and Oxford: Princeton University Press.

Bishop, P. (1995). *The Dionysian Self: C. G. Jung's Reception of Friedrich Nietzsche*. Berlin and New York: Walter de Gruyter.

Bishop, P. (2008). *Analytical Psychology and German Classical Aesthetics: Goethe, Schiller, and Jung: The Development of Personality* (Vol. 1). London and New York: Routledge.

Bishop, P. (2009). *Analytical Psychology and German Classical Aesthetics: Goethe, Schiller, and Jung: The Constellation of the Self* (Vol. 2). London and New York: Routledge.

Bradotti, R. (2012). 'Nomadic ethics'. In D. W. Smith and H. Somers-Hall (Eds.), *The Cambridge Companion to Deleuze*, 170–97. Cambridge: Cambridge University Press.

Colebrook, C. (2010). *Deleuze and the Meaning of Life*. London and New York: Continuum Press.

Conley, T. (2005). Noology. In A. Parr (Ed.), *The Deleuze Dictionary*, 165–66. Edinburgh: Edinburgh University Press.

Delanda, M. (2009). Assemblages against totalities. In H. Berressem and L. Haferkamp (Eds.), *Deleuzian Events: Writing History*, 34–42. Münster: Lit Verlag.

Deleuze, G. (1966/2000). *Proust and Signs* (R. Howard, Trans.). Minneapolis: University of Minnesota Press.

Deleuze, G. (1968/1994). *Difference and Repetition* (P. Patton, Trans.). New York: Columbia University Press.

Deleuze, G. (1981/2003). *Francis Bacon: The Logic of Sensation* (D. W. Smith, Trans.). Minneapolis, MN: University of Minnesota Press.

Deleuze, G. (1983/1986). *Cinema 1: The Movement-Image* (H. Tomlinson and B. Habberjam, Trans.). Minneapolis: University of Minnesota.

Deleuze, G. (1985/1989). *Cinema 2: The Time-Image* (H. Tomlinson and R. Galeta, Trans.). Minneapolis: University of Minnesota.

Deleuze, G., and Guattari, F (1972/1983). *Anti-Oedipus: Capitalism and Schizophrenia* (R. Hurley, M. Seem and H. R. Lane, Trans.). Minneapolis: University of Minnesota Press.

Deleuze, G., and Guattari, F. (1986). *Kafka: Towards a Minor Literature* (D. Polan, Trans.). Minneapolis: University of Minnesota Press.

Deleuze, G., and Guattari, F (1980/1987). *A Thousand Plateaus: Capitalism and Schizophrenia* (B. Massumi, Trans.). Minneapolis: University of Minnesota Press.

Deleuze, G., and Guattari, F (1991/1994). *What is Philosophy?* (H. Tomlinson and G. Burchell, Trans.). New York: Columbia University Press.

Homans, P. (1995). *Jung in Context: Modernity and the Making of a Psychology*. Chicago and London: University of Chicago Press.

Jung, C. G. (1899). Thoughts on the interpretation of Christianity, with reference to the theory of Albrecht Ritschl. In *The Collected Works of C. G. Jung* (Sir H. Read, M. Fordham, and G. Adler, Eds.; W. McGuire, Exec. Ed.;

R. F. C. Hull, Trans.) [hereafter *Collected Works*], Supplementary Vol. A, *The Zofingia Lectures* (J. Van Heurck, Trans.), 93–111. London: Routledge.

Jung, C. G. (1921). *Collected Works,* vol. 6, *Psychological Types.* London: Routledge & Kegan Paul, 1969.

Jung, C. G. (1930/1950). Psychology and literature. In *Collected Works*, vol. 15, *The Spirit in Man, Art, and Literature*, 84–105. London: Routledge & Kegan Paul, 1966.

Jung, C. G. (1934). The practical use of dream-analysis. In *Collected Works,* vol. 16, *The Practice of Psychotherapy*, 2nd ed., 139–61. London: Routledge & Kegan Paul, 1966.

Jung, C. G. (1936/1954). Concerning the archetypes, with special reference to the anima concept. In *Collected Works,* vol. 9i, *The Archetypes and the Collective Unconscious*, 2nd ed., 54–72. London: Routledge & Kegan Paul, 1969.

Jung, C. G. (1938/1940). Psychology and religion. In *Collected Works,* vol. 11, *Psychology and Religion: West and East*, 2nd ed. London: Routledge & Kegan Paul, 1969.

Jung, C. G. (1939). Conscious, unconscious, and individuation. In *Collected Works,* vol. 9i, *The Archetypes and the Collective Unconscious*, 2nd ed., 279–85. London: Routledge & Kegan Paul, 1969.

Jung, C. G. (1945). Psychotherapy today. In *Collected Works,* vol. 16, *The Practice of Psychotherapy*, 2nd ed., 94–110. London: Routledge & Kegan Paul, 1966.

Jung, C. G. (1947/1954). On the nature of the psyche. In *Collected Works,* vol. 8, *The Structure and Dynamics of the Psyche*, 2nd ed., 159–234. London: Routledge & Kegan Paul, 1969.

Jung, C. G. (1957). The undiscovered self (present and future). In *Collected Works,* vol. 10, *Civilisation in Transition*, 2nd ed., 245–305. London: Routledge & Kegan Paul, 1963.

Kerslake, C. (2004). Rebirth through incest. *Angelaki* 9(1): 135–57.

Kerslake, C. (2007). *Deleuze and the Unconscious.* London and New York: Continuum Press.

Lambert, G. (2003). *The Non-Philosophy of Gilles Deleuze.* London and New York: Continuum Press.

Lambert, G. (2012). *In Search of a New Image of Thought: Gilles Deleuze and Philosophical Expressionism.* Minneapolis and London: University of Minnesota Press.

Main, R. (2004). *The Rupture of Time: Synchronicity and Jung's Critique of Modern Western Culture.* Hove and New York: Brunner-Routledge.

McGrath, S. (2014). The question concerning metaphysics: A Schellingian intervention in analytical psychology. *International Journal of Jungian Studies* 6(1): 23–51.

Patton, P. (2000). *Deleuze and the Political.* London and New York: Routledge.

Patton, P. (2012). Deleuze's Political Philosophy. In D. Smith and H. Somers-Hall (Eds.), *The Cambridge Companion to Deleuze*, 198–219. Cambridge: Cambridge University Press.

Toscano, A. (2006). *The Theatre of Production: Philosophy and Individuation between Kant and Deleuze.* Basingstoke and New York: Palgrave Macmillan.

Chapter 3

Jung as symptomatologist

David Henderson

Reading Deleuze, one *hears* Jung. The internal resonance between Jung's psychological theory and Deleuze's philosophy is uncanny. Žižek (2004) in characteristically pithy fashion states: 'No wonder, then, that an admiration of Jung is Deleuze's corpse in the closet; the fact that Deleuze borrowed a key term (*rhizome*) from Jung is not a mere insignificant accident – rather, it points toward a deeper link' (ibid.: 662). This deeper link has been more sympathetically explored by Kerslake (2002, 2004, 2006, 2007, 2009), Semetsky (2004, 2006; Lovat and Semetsky 2009; Semetsky and Delpech-Ramey 2012), McMillan (2012, 2018), and Jenkins (2016). They provide us with the only systematic studies of Deleuze and Jung available thus far. This chapter is part of an interest in using concepts from the work of Deleuze to amplify elements of Jung's theory. In this case, it employs the concepts of symptomatology, percept and minor literature from Deleuze's discussion of the critical and the clinical. As such, it belongs to Jungian studies rather than constituting an intervention in Deleuzian philosophy. It is preliminary spadework, experimental exploration of the rhizome, rather than definitive interpretation.

Deleuze introduced the theme of the critical and the clinical in his 1967 essay, 'Coldness and cruelty', an analysis of the concept of sadomasochism, arguing that 'The critical (in the literary sense) and the clinical (in the medical sense) may be destined to enter into a new relationship of mutual learning' (Deleuze 1991: 14). He suggested that, 'Because the judgement of the clinician is prejudiced we must take an entirely different approach, the *literary approach*, since it is from literature that stem the original definitions of sadism and masochism' (ibid.). The diagnostic power of literature continued to be a preoccupation for

Deleuze up to his final book, *Essays Critical and Clinical* (1997a), first published in 1993.

His interest however is avowedly philosophical, not literary or clinical. Deleuze (2014) insists that 'A philosophical concept can never be confused with a scientific function or an artistic construction, but finds itself in *affinity* with these in this or that domain of science or style of art' (ibid.: xiii). Philosophy exploits these affinities for its own purposes. It 'always enters into relations of mutual resonance and exchange with these other domains for reasons that are always internal to philosophy itself' (Smith 1997: xii).

Does Deleuze's project of the critical and the clinical resonate in the rhizome of psychoanalysis? Freud (1925) said that psychoanalysis is located between philosophy and medicine. Jung's (1989) description of his decision to specialise in psychiatry points to similarly liminal territory:

> Here alone the two currents of my interest could flow together and in a united stream dig their own bed. Here was the empirical field common to biological and spiritual facts, which I had everywhere sought and nowhere found. Here at last was the place where the collision of nature and spirit became a reality.
>
> (Jung 1989: 109)

Psychoanalysis wrestles with the angel of inbetweenness. It is not entirely one thing or another. Is it science or is it hermeneutics? Is it knowledge or is it narrative?

Among these uncertainties, there is the constant tension in psychoanalytic theory and practice between what is internal to the session or the analysis and influences or pressures coming from outside of the clinical frame. Like Deleuze's philosophy, psychoanalysis wants to engage in these relations of mutual resonance and exchange with neighbouring discourses for reasons that are internal to itself. It is ultimately concerned with resolving its own clinical and theoretical dilemmas, and not necessarily with shedding new light on other areas of knowledge. There is an ethical debate within the profession between those who prioritise clinical experience and those who give greater relative weight to concepts and demands coming from outside of the clinical domain. For example, there are those who argue that it is essential for psychoanalysts to be knowledgeable about neuroscience and those who feel that neuroscience has nothing of significance to contribute to our understanding of the analytic process. Infant observation is another example. Some trainings require students to undertake a two-year infant observation in order to understand the developmental process in depth. Others take the approach that there is not necessarily a correspondence between the historical baby and the child archetype, or between the observed infant and the clinical infant, as Stern (1985) has described them. Similarly, Hillman (1964) argues that the meaning of suicide within psychoanalysis is radically different from the significance it carries in other disciplines such as sociology, medicine, law or religion. This controversy extends to the reverse direction as well, to the long-standing discussion about the status of applied psychoanalysis, where it is debated to what extent concepts generated in clinical experience are applicable to the world outside the clinic.

In all of these cases it can be argued that ultimately the usefulness or purpose of exploring the affinities, resonances and exchanges with extra-analytic domains arises from reasons internal to analysis itself. We can hear an echo here of Jung's insistence that he was approaching issues and questions as a psychologist – not as a philosopher or theologian. He was alert to an astonishing range of adjacent discourses and he was adept at enlisting concepts from these disparate fields for his own purposes.

Symptomatology

Deleuze identified three key features of medicine: symptomatology, etiology and therapy. Syptomatology is the study of signs. Etiology is the search for causes. Therapy is the development and application of a treatment. According to Smith (1997), 'While etiology and therapeutics are integral parts of medicine, symptomatology appeals to a kind of limit-point, premedical or submedical, that belongs as much to art as to medicine' (ibid.: xvi). Deleuze (1983) aligns his concept of symptomatology with Nietzsche's active science, as opposed to a passive, reactive or negative science. 'A *symptomatology* [...] interprets phenomena, treating them as symptoms whose sense must be sought in the forces that produce them' (ibid.: 70). This critique is productive. As Kaiser (2017) observes, 'Symptoms are perspectival and subjective [...]. Symptomatology is used as a critical tool, an activity to distil the relations of forces underlying the currently congealed order of things' (ibid.: 185–86). 'The point of critique is not justification but a different way of feeling: another sensitivity' (Deleuze 1983: 88).

Illnesses are often identified with the names of the scientists who isolated a constellation of symptoms or the names of patients who suffered from the syndrome – for example, Lou Gehrig's disease, Parkinson's disease, Roger's disease, Alzheimer's disease, or Cruetzfeldt-Jakob's disease. Deleuze (1990) argued that literary figures, among them Lewis Carol, Zola, Fitzgerald, Artaud, Kafka, Proust and Beckett, are symptomatologists, readers of signs. He was interested in these writers, not as patients, but as 'clinicians of civilization':

> Authors, if they are great, are more like doctors than patients. We mean that they are themselves astonishing diagnosticians or symptomatologists. There is always a great deal of art involved in the grouping of symptoms, in the organization of a *table* (*tableau*) where a particular symptom is dissociated from another, juxtaposed to a third, and forms the new figure of a disorder or illness. Clinicians who are able to renew a symtomatological picture produce a work of art; conversely, artists are clinicians, not with respect to their own case, nor even with respect to a case in general; rather, they are clinicians of civilization.
>
> (Deleuze 1990: 237)

For Jung (1966), art performs critical, interpretive and regulative functions:

> Therein lies the social significance of art: it is constantly at work educating the spirit of the age, conjuring up the forms in which the age is most lacking [...] so art represents a process of self-regulation in the life of nations and epochs.
>
> (ibid.: pars. 130–31)

A good deal of psychoanalytic literary criticism produces what are in essence case studies that use clinical concepts to analyse the psychopathology of authors, their plots and characters. Jung (1993a) was critical of this approach:

> [I]t is sometimes possible to explain a work of art in the same way as one can explain a nervous illness in terms of Freud's theory or Adler's. But when it comes to great poetry the pathological explanation, the attempt to apply Freudian or Adlerian theory, is in effect a ridiculous belittlement of the work of art. The explanation not only contributes nothing to an understanding of the poetry, but, on the contrary, deflects our gaze from that deeper vision which the poet offers. [...] great art is man's creation of something superhuman in defiance of all the ordinary, miserable conditions of his birth and childhood. To apply to this the psychology of neurosis is little short of grotesque.
>
> (Jung 1993a: pars. 1723–24)

However, Deleuze (1990) argues that Freud also functioned as a symptomatologist: 'From the perspective of Freud's genius, it is not the complex which provides us with information about Oedipus and Hamlet, but rather Oedipus and Hamlet who provide us with information about the complex' (ibid.: 237). It is Oedipus and Hamlet who illuminate the suffering of the patient, not a putatively neutral or objective, clinical concept. Freud 'discovered' the Oedipus complex by exploiting literature to organise certain clinical phenomena.

It is symptomatology that opens the door for Deleuze (2004) into psychoanalysis and psychiatry:

> I would never have permitted myself to write on psychoanalysis and psychiatry were I not dealing with the problem of symptomatology. Symptomatology is situated almost outside of medicine, at a neutral point, a zero point, where artists and philosophers and doctors and patients can encounter each other.
>
> (Deleuze 2004: 134)

It seems natural that we would find Jung in that encounter of artists, philosophers, doctors and patients. What can we learn about Jung if we think of him as a symptomatologist? How can Deleuze amplify our understanding of Jung? Is Jung like a novelist 'who invents unknown or unrecognized affects and brings them to light as the becoming of his characters' (Deleuze and Guattari 1994: 174)?

Symptomatology functions in terms of the proper name and the 'multiplicity' or 'assemblage' that is referred to. Jung's name is often associated with certain clinical phenomena, we could say assemblages, such as Jungian complexes, Jungian archetypes, the Jungian collective unconscious, Jungian analysis, Jungian analyst, Jungian dreams, Jungian self. In each of these cases Jung has drawn together certain psychic phenomena and organised particular constellations of experience. New relations between psychic elements are brought to light and can be discussed. To label these as Jungian is both meaningful and meaningless. The label simultaneously illuminates and obscures. The very name of Jung informs us and blinds us. While he has brought to light striking new psychological facts, the aura of 'Jung' in the minds of some of his followers can eclipse the very phenomena with which he was experimenting.

Deleuze argues that literary artists, through the act of writing, reveal life, a life, non-organic life. 'In reality *writing does not have its end in itself, precisely because life is not something personal*. Or rather, the aim of writing is to carry life to the state of a non-personal power' (Deleuze and Parnet 1987: 50). Gesturing toward a similar theme in Jung's writing, Rowland (2005) observes:

> Jung offers the notion of the 'symbol' in which the work or image is an emblem of the unknown or unknowable. Such art principally speaks a language foreign to the ego of its author; its significance surpasses traces of the formation of the ego. Such art is autonomous of the author because it is rooted in the *collective* unconscious, not reliant upon the author's *personal* life, but rather his *impersonal one.* For symbolic art, the author is not a guide to the work.
>
> (Rowland 2005: 8)

Rowland highlights the compensatory function of art in Jung's theory: 'Such art represents the healing self-regulation of the psyche amplified into the cultural dimension [...] symbolic art structurally transforms collective culture in ways that amount to an internal self-regulating mechanism' (ibid.: 11).

For Deleuze, the question that a literary work poses is not 'What does it mean?' but rather 'How does it function?' The work does not propose interpretations. It evokes experimentation. The literary machine is made up of fragments, singularities. The work of art is to 'establish a system of communication among these parts or elements that are in themselves noncommunicating' (Smith 1997: xxiii). It produces a unity of parts, but it does not unify the parts:

> [T]he whole produced by the work is rather a 'peripheral' totality that is added *alongside* its parts as a *new* singularity fabricated separately. [...] The work thus constitutes a whole, but this whole is itself a part that merely exists alongside the other parts, which it neither unifies nor totalizes. Yet it nonetheless has an *effect* on these parts, since it is able to create nonpreexistent relations between elements that in themselves remain disconnected, and are left intact. [...] the Whole is never a principle but rather an effect [...]. The Whole, in other words, is the Open, because it is its nature to constantly produce or create the *new*.
>
> (Smith 1997: xxiii)

The suggestion that in this particular notion of the whole the elements 'in themselves remain disconnected, and are left intact' resonates with Cusa's (1997) statement that the coincidence of opposites is a 'unity to which neither otherness nor plurality nor multiplicity is opposed' (ibid.: 121). The coincidence of opposites is one of Jung's key images of the whole (Henderson 2014). To the extent that Jung follows Cusa, this is a whole that does not extinguish difference or singularity. The assertion that the nature of Deleuze's 'whole' is 'to constantly produce or create the new' echoes Jung (1959c), who argues that 'one should not overlook the fact that in reality man's procreative power is only a special instance of the "procreative nature of the Whole"' (ibid.: par. 313).

There are some immediate applications of these thoughts to Jung's view of individuation. They give us a way of thinking about the experiment of individuation as something that produces a sense of wholeness that exists alongside the many elements of the personality and the unconscious. It promotes communication between the elements without subordinating them to a greater identity. We could say that therapy is about discovering possibilities, differences, rather than producing a monolithic personality structure. As Searles notes (Sedgwick 1993), individuation increases the capacity to live with multiplicity; it does not iron things out. Jung's (1959a) wry observation that 'Were it not for the leaping and twinkling of the soul, man would rot away in his greatest passion, idleness' (ibid.: par. 56) resonates with the idea that it is the function of literature to stir us to experimentation and to enable communication between fragments and singularities. Like Jung's 'leaping and twinkling of the soul', Deleuze (1983) characterises Nietzsche's will to power as '*essentially creative and giving*: it does not aspire, it does not seek, it does not desire, above all it does not desire power. It *gives*: power is something inexpressible in the will (something mobile, variable, plastic); power is in the will as "the bestowing virtue", through power the will itself bestows sense and value' (ibid.: 80).

Deleuze's primary concern in his thinking about literature is Life, non-organic life. In an interview he stated: 'You have seen what is essential for me, this "vitalism" or a conception of life as a non-organic power' (Smith 1997: xiii). Writing is the vehicle that is able 'to carry life to the state of a non-personal power' (Deleuze and Parnet 1987: 50). Deleuze refers to a scene in Charles Dickens's *Our Mutual Friend* about a man, despised by everyone, who is on his deathbed:

> No one has the least regard for the man. With them all, he has been an object of avoidance, suspicion, and aversion; but the spark of life within him is curiously separate from himself now, and they have a deep interest in it, probably because it is life, and they are living and must die.
>
> (Dickens 1952: 443)

Deleuze observes something similar in babies:

> Small infants all resemble each other and have hardly any individuality; but they have singularities – a smile, a gesture, a grimace – which are not subjective characteristics. Infants are transversed by an immanent life that is pure power, and even a beatitude through their sufferings and weakness.
>
> (Deleuze 2001: 30)

It is fair to say that analysts are – or should be – acutely attuned to these sparks, singularities and spontaneous gestures. You might call these experiences encounters with the archetypal aspect of existence. They are pre-personal, transpersonal and post-personal. You could see them as experiences of the Jungian self. Dickens's character and Deleuze's infant resonate with Jung's (1993b) description of the 'collective level' of experience:

> Because the basic structure of the mind is the same in everybody, we cannot make distinctions when we experience on that level. There we do not know if something has happened to you or to me. In the underlying collective level there is a wholeness which cannot be dissected. If you begin to think about participation as a fact which means that fundamentally we are identical with everybody and everything, you are led to very peculiar theoretical conclusions. You should not go further than those conclusions because these things get dangerous. But some of the conclusions you should explore, because they can explain a lot of peculiar things that happen to man.
>
> (Jung 1993b: par. 87)

These experiences have peculiar and possibly dangerous effects on our minds. They are present in the dying man and the newborn infant:

> In this idea the all-embracing nature of psychic wholeness is expressed. Wholeness is never comprised within the compass of the conscious mind – it includes the indefinite and indefinable extent of the unconscious as well. Wholeness, empirically speaking, is therefore of immeasurable extent, older and younger than consciousness and enfolding it in time and space.
>
> (Jung 1959b: par. 299)

One thing that the dying man and the newborn infant have in common is a lack of cognitive capacity and self-consciousness. Non-organic life is witnessed by the people assembled at the deathbed and by the baby's parents. As Jung (1959c) says, the conscious mind can only have a tenuous awareness of wholeness: 'Empirically speaking, consciousness can never comprehend the whole, but it is probable that the whole is unconsciously present in the ego' (ibid.: par. 171).

Jung maintained that Christ is an archetypal image of the self in a Western context. Is witnessing non-organic life akin to seeing god in one's neighbour?

> The spontaneous symbols of the self, or of wholeness, cannot in practice be distinguished from a God-image. [...] there is an ever-present archetype of wholeness which may easily disappear from the purview of consciousness or may never be perceived at all.
>
> (ibid.: par. 73)

It could be argued that Mother Teresa had a vocation to witness signs of this non-organic life in the dying people she nursed on the streets of Kolkata.

According to Jung (1956), 'When an idea is so old and so generally believed, it must be true in some way, by which I mean that it is *psychologically true*' (ibid.: par. 4). Is it *psychologically true* that non-organic life *is* wholeness? Did Jung acting as a symptomatologist diagnose the vicissitudes of non-organic life in the domain of human experience? He wrote about the perils of lack of contact with this life and of over-identification with it. He was concerned with how to establish a viable relationship with wholeness.

A viable relationship with non-organic life or wholeness involves a combination of openness and resilience:

> Literature then appears as an enterprise of health: not that the writer would necessarily be in good health [...] but he possesses an irresistible and delicate health that stems from what he has seen and heard of things too big for him, too strong for him, suffocating things whose passage exhausts him, while nonetheless giving him the becomings that his dominant and substantial health would render impossible.
>
> (Deleuze 1997b: 228)

Often the popular notion of the wounded healer implies that there is trauma in the therapist's past that they have dealt with or confronted in their own therapy, and that this informs the therapist's engagement with clients or patients in the present. Deleuze's construction raises the question as to whether the practice of psychotherapy is in itself damaging, wounding, shaming and debilitating for the therapist. The resilient therapist is not an invulnerable therapist. As Freud (1930) observed, 'Life, as we find it, is too hard for us; it brings us too many pains, disappointments, and impossible tasks' (ibid.: 75).

Percept

The percept is a type of *vision* or *hearing*. Are there particular features in the way that Jung saw and heard that contributed to his position as a symptomatologist? François Zourabichvili (1996) describes the percept as 'A critical-clinical perception. *Critical* because we discern a force in it, a particular type of force, and *clinical* because we evaluate the declination of this force, its inclination, its ability to fold or unfold itself' (ibid.: 192). The percept is one of five themes in Deleuze's work that are important to the critical and clinical project as described by Smith (1997): 1) the destruction of the world (Singularities and Events); 2) the dissolution of the subject (Affects and Percepts); 3) the dis-integration of the body (Intensities and Becomings); 4) the 'minorization' of politics (Speech Acts and Fabulations); 5) the 'stuttering' of language (Syntax and Style).

The theme of the dissolution of the subject has affinities with Jung's confrontation with the unconscious, in which he encountered spontaneous and autonomous images and affects. He discovered the landscape of the collective unconscious. In grappling with these experiences, he formulated his theories out of unknown and unrecognised forces. As Deleuze observes: 'A great novelist is above all an artist who invents unknown or unrecognized affects and brings them to light as the becoming of his characters' (Deleuze and Guattari 1994: 174). Jung's 'characters' are the archetypes, archetypal images, and a distinctive approach to clinical practice. The disturbing impact of the percept is a basic component in the formation of concepts:

> It is independent of the creator through the self-positing of the created, which is preserved in itself. What is preserved – the thing or the work of art – is *a bloc of sensations, that is to say, a compound*

of percepts and affects. Percepts are no longer perceptions; they are independent of a state of those who experience them. Affects are no longer feelings or affections; they go beyond the strength of those who undergo them. Sensations, percepts, and affects are *beings* whose validity lies in themselves and exceeds any lived.

(Deleuze and Guattari 1994: 164)

Beginning with his confrontation with the unconscious, Jung refined his vision and hearing by working with his patients and on the *Red Book*. He was interested in the autonomous unconscious, whose contents 'are independent of a state of those who experience them'. According to Zourabichvili (1996), 'Deleuze is less concerned to fix an essence of the appearing of things, than with bringing out and differentiating the *non-organic life* that they involve' (ibid.: 191).

This points to a tension in analytical psychology between a wish to interpret archetypes and archetypal images and a wish to experiment with them; a tendency to fix the essence of an image and a tendency to be sensitive to the non-organic life, the wholeness in the image. This can appear as a choice between viewing the archetypal image as a representation of the archetype or viewing the archetypal image as the site of archetypal pressure. To ask of Jung 'What were you thinking of?' could be rephrased as 'What did you see?' or better, 'How did you see?'

How does sight regain its power when it becomes vision, or percept? When one sees the *invisible*, the *imperceptible*, or when what cannot be seen is perceived: the invisible enveloped in what one sees, not as a hidden world beyond appearance, but animating sight itself from within appearance, or what one sees […] it is necessary that the invisible seen is the invisible *of* the visible itself, the 'being of the sensible'.

(Zourabichvili 1996: 190)

Was Jung interested in the invisible of the visible or was he interested in a hidden world? Without a doubt many of his disciples take up his work as a description and exploration of a hidden world. Much of his work lends itself to that sort of interpretation, but it can be argued that in his writings on the practice of psychotherapy he is attending to the invisible of the visible. This resonates with Winnicott's plea that the mother must see the baby that is really there, not the baby that she might wish for, or fear, or feel is expected of her. Can the therapist see the non-organic life, the wholeness, in the patient?

What sort of experience did Jung have that enabled him to formulate his picture of a new landscape – the collective unconscious? As Zourabichvili (1996) observes, 'To live a landscape: one is no longer in front of it, but in it, one passes into the landscape' (ibid.: 196). When Jung's inner landscape came alive and he entered the drama, his relationship with the unconscious changed. He was no longer observing memories and representations. He became an actor and he was acted upon. He was no longer observing the soul, but living with soul. The expanse and force of this newly discovered landscape placed a demand on him as a writer. Jung discusses this in terms of excess libido:

> This excess libido constitutes the essential precondition to developing a culture [...]. As such, the symbol is also the *mother of science* [...] 'initiating' a sustained playful interest in the object that allows man to make all sorts of discoveries which would otherwise have escaped him [...]
>
> (Gieser 2014: 153)

In his confrontation with the unconscious, Jung experienced visions and intuitions that threw him into turmoil. As Zourabichvili observes, 'Can we speak of a profound landscape, as we say of an idea? An idea is not profound because it is well-founded, in close contact with its foundations, but rather because it makes thought 'founder' [*effondant*] and liberates the infinite resonances in chaotic communication within it' (1996: 200). Similarly, Jung's concepts presuppose a collapse in the face of the unknown. Zourabichvili again:

> The writer, far from reporting lived experience, makes a vital discovery. He sees at the limit of the livable, he lives what cannot be lived through. [...] Deleuze appears to give two reasons, two arguments for the idea that the percept exceeds all lived experience and exists in the absence of man: (1) it overflows subjectivity, and (2) it conserves itself independently of that which experiences it and

composes it. So, he specifies, it is a matter of a conservation *in itself* (and not only in some material).

(Zourabichvili 1996: 201)

Jung's (1964) percept, the collective unconscious, is autonomous and it 'was psyche long before there was any ego conscious, and will remain psyche no matter how far our ego consciousness extends' (ibid.: par. 304).

The *Red Book* represents, among other things, Jung's attempt to grapple with the expanse and force of this newly discovered landscape. He is wrestling with personal and collective turbulence. The *Red Book* contains a number of features, which can be taken as evidence for the view that Jung can be read as a symptomatologist. According to Beebe (2014), the book is:

> a living memorial to the psychological experience of surviving the disorientation occasioned by the emergence of [...] a 'psychic epidemic', the affects associated with the arrival of World War I [...]. [It] dramatizes with skill not only the abreaction of the fragmented psychic state of one individual traumatized by historical upheaval, but also the therapeutic strategies for self-healing that can emerge out of such an experience. The *Red Book* thus provides in literary form a model of how the integrity of psyche can be restored in the face of cultural processes that threaten to undermine it.
>
> (Beebe 2014: 108–9)

Beebe identifies the *Red Book* as a 'trickster work of art' fuelled by rage at Freud and the psychoanalytic movement (ibid.: 109). Although Beebe doesn't explicitly say so, the inference can be drawn that this personal rage resonates with the rage unleashed by World War I. Beebe argues that the book tells a 'post-heroic story' (ibid.: 113). The demand to discover a post-heroic approach is raised by Jung's own mid-life dilemmas, as well as by the need to recognise the limitations of rationality in culture and politics:

> The times were demanding, as if from within themselves, that the heroic quest for a brilliant adaptation be sacrificed [...]. This time,

its direction is not up toward mastery, but down into a profound acceptance of incapacity.

(ibid.: 114)

In the face of hubris and the striving toward rational perfection, on a personal *or* a collective level, Jung, as symptomatologist, prescribes the experience of limitation and learning 'how to hold one's capacity in tension with one's incapacity' (ibid.: 116).

As a symptomatologist, Jung diagnoses the failures of psychology and psychotherapy. '*The Red Book*', writes Sanford Drob, 'can be metaphorically understood as a dream, not the dream of an individual person, but the dream of the discipline and practice of psychology' (Drob 2012: 260). In the face of the tendency to understand 'the psychotherapeutic process in simple cognitive, pragmatic, and manualized terms, [Jung] reminds us that psychological exploration has the potential to open worlds as well as treat symptoms' (ibid.: 263). The *Red Book* is an expression of Jung's experiment with wholeness. According to Hogenson (2014), 'The *Red Book* is Jung's umwelt, and, as such, it represents Jung's recovery of the holistic image in the age of the sciences' (ibid.: 104).

Minor literature

The minorisation of politics and minor literature are further elements of Deleuze's thought about the critical and the clinical that can be used to amplify Jung's own writings and the work of analytical psychologists as minor literature. In their discussion of Kafka and minor literature, Deleuze and Guattari (1986) observe:

A minor literature doesn't come from a minor language; it is rather that which a minority constructs within a major language. But the first characteristic of minor literature in any case is that in it language is affected with a high coefficient of deterritorialization. [...] In short, Prague German is a deterritorialized language, appropriate for strange and minor uses.

(Deleuze and Guattari 1986: 16–17)

Jung was adept at appropriating the language of science, psychology, religion and philosophy for his own 'strange' uses. He is 'a foreigner *within* his own language' (Bogue 2003: 100). This may account for some of the bewilderment and hostility expressed toward Jung's work. Like Kafka, he has taken familiar words and images and infused them with destabilising intent:

> Kafka's Yiddish [...] is not so much a language as a way of inhabiting language, a minority's means of appropriating the majority's tongue and undermining its fixed structure. Yiddish speakers, like Prague Jews, make a *minor* use of language, a destabilising deformation of the standard elements of German that sets it in motion and opens it to forces of metamorphosis.
>
> (Bogue 2003: 97)

The sometime kaleidoscopic and florid impression that Jung's writing gives can be seen as an aspect of the experimental nature of his thought. People can feel at sea in the *Collected Works*. As Bogue (2003) observes, this resonates with the view of Deleuze and Guattari that:

> to invent something new is necessarily to invent something whose shape cannot be foreseen. The new emerges through a process of metamorphosis whose outcome is unpredictable. If writers find existing configurations of social relations unacceptable, their only option is to induce a metamorphosis of the established forms of the social field, with no guarantee that the result will be a more acceptable community. It is for this reason that in a minor literature expression precedes content: "it is expression that outdistances or advances, it is expression that precedes contents."
>
> (Bogue 2003: 110)

Jung was led by his dreams, visions, active imagination, intuition, sculpture and play toward the formation of his own language. A major literature starts from given content, whereas minor literature starts with expression:

> A major, or established, literature follows a vector that goes from content to expression. Since content is presented in a given form of the content, one must find, discover, or see the form of expression that goes with it. [...] But minor, or revolutionary, literature

begins by expressing itself and doesn't conceptualise until after-
ward. [...] Expression must break forms, encourage ruptures and
new sproutings.

(Deleuze and Guattari 1986: 28)

The notion of a minor literature has a political dimension. It is not
the creation of an individual and is not dominated by a towering figure. A hagiographic attitude toward Jung can obscure the collective
nature of his work. As Bogue (2003) states:

In the absence of a people, writers who are marginalized and solitary may be in the best position "to express another potential community", but if they do so, it will not be as individual subjects, for
"the most individual literary enunciation is a particular case of
collective enunciation".

(Bogue 2003: 111)

As a solitary explorer of the psyche, Jung had rhizomatic links with
others contributing to a common endeavour:

It is here that we confront Deleuze's conception of the political
destiny of literature. Just as writers do not write with their egos,
neither do they write "on behalf of" an already existing people or
"address" themselves to a class or nation. [...] what they find rather
is that "the people are missing."

(Smith 1997: xli)

The writer is part of the creation of a people. Literature has the
capacity to create a nation. This idea has uncanny resonances with
Zeller's (1975) description of his discussion with Jung about a dream:

Dream: *A temple of vast dimensions was in the process of being
built. As far as I could see – ahead, behind, right and left – there were
incredible numbers of people building on gigantic pillars. I, too, was
building on a pillar. The whole building process was in its very first
beginnings, but the foundation was already there, the rest of the building was starting to go up, and I and many others were working on it.*

Jung said, 'Ja, you know, that is the temple we all build on. We don't know the people because, believe me, they build in India and China and in Russia and all over the world. That is the new religion. You know how long it will take until it is built?'

I said, 'How should I know? Do you know?'

He said, 'I know.'

I asked how long it will take.

He said, 'About six hundred years.'

'Where do you know this from?' I asked.

He said, 'From dreams. From other people's dreams and from my own. This new religion will come together as far as we can see.'

(Zeller 1975: 2)

Whether this story demonstrates Jung's supreme confidence in his own interpretations of the unconscious or his experiments in the rhizome of dreams I am not sure, but it resonates with Deleuze's approach in that both the writer and the dreamer are contributing to the creation of new political and cultural formations.

As a consequence of Jung's prescription of holism as the remedy for the personal, cultural, ethical and religious ills that assail modern Western civilisation, it could be argued that he initiated a minor literature and a minority politics. In the world of psychoanalytic writing, analytical psychology is a minor literature and within the professional world of psychoanalysis, Jungian associations practice minority politics. As Be Pannell explains:

Minor literature is characterised by a concern not with concepts developed by individual subjects at the centre of literary action, but rather what is given to perception; the forces encountered by the body, experienced as intensities, percepts and affects from which concepts are constructed. This has important implications for psychology, as minor literature articulates modes of becoming that do not emphasise the individual subject. These intensities, percepts and affects are fleeting and non-representable, where every form that takes shape at infinite speeds vanishes as soon as it appears.

(Pannell 2018: 196)

Jung's writings on psychotherapy are saturated with references to the 'fleeting and non-representable', the limits of the analyst's understanding, the plasticity of the psyche and the fluidity of the analytic process (Henderson 2014). It might be argued that the liminality of the practice, theory and institutions of analytical psychology is central to the potency of its creative contribution to psychoanalysis. One is reminded of the centrality of the inferior function in Jung's thought. While there is pressure to bring analytical psychology to a more established position, it may be worth considering the words of Deleuze and Guattari (1983): 'Only the minor is great and revolutionary' (ibid.: 26).

Conclusion

This chapter began with the assertion that 'Reading Deleuze, one *hears* Jung'. It has explored possible resonances between Jung's psychology and Deleuze's philosophy as a way of amplifying our appreciation of analytical psychology. It has made use of Deleuze's concepts of symptomatology, percept and minor literature, from his writings on the critical and the clinical. As a symptomatologist, Jung can be seen as a 'clinician of civilization', who discovered the collective unconscious and prescribed a renewed relationship with wholeness as a remedy for the personal, cultural and collective dis-eases of modern life. The percept is a type of *vision* and *hearing*. Jung's encounter with elements of the autonomous unconscious engendered turbulence, which stimulated the production of the *Red Book* and the articulation of new theories and clinical methodologies. Jung's writing can be read as a minor literature which destabilises the language of psychoanalysis and psychology for 'strange and minor uses' and the institutions of analytical psychology can be understood as practising minority politics in the world of psychoanalysis. There is ample scope for further experimentation with the thought of Deleuze to illuminate the texture of the rhizome of analytical psychology.

Acknowledgement

Work on this chapter was supported by the Arts and Humanities Research Council [AH/N003853/1].

References

Beebe, J. (2014). *The Red Book* as a work of literature. In T. Kirsch and G. Hogenson (Eds.), *The Red Book: Reflections on C. G. Jung's Liber Novus*, 108–22. London: Routledge.

Bogue, R. (2003). *Deleuze on Literature*. London: Routledge.

Buchanan, I. (2006). Deleuze's 'life' sentences. *Polygraph: An International Journal of Culture and Politics*, *18*: 129–47.

Cusa, N. (1997). On learned ignorance. In *Selected Spiritual Writings* (H. L. Bond, Trans.), 85–206. Mahwah, NJ: Paulist Press.

Deleuze, G. (1983). *Nietzsche and Philosophy*. London: Bloomsbury.

Deleuze, G. (1990). *Logic of Sense*. New York: Columbia University Press.

Deleuze, G. (1991). *Masochism*. New York: Zone Books.

Deleuze, G. (1997a). *Essays Critical and Clinical*. Minneapolis: University of Minnesota Press.

Deleuze, G. (1997b). Literature and life. *Critical Inquiry*, *23*(2): 225–30.

Deleuze, G. (2001). *Pure Immanence: Essays on a Life*. New York: Zone Books.

Deleuze, G. (2004). *Desert Islands and Other Texts* (S. Lotinger, Ed.; M. Taormina, Trans.). New York: Semiotext(e).

Deleuze, G. (2014). *Difference and Repetition*. London: Bloomsbury.

Deleuze, G., and Guattari, F. (1983). What is a minor literature? *Mississippi Review*, *11*(3), 13–33.

Deleuze, G., and Guattari, F. (1986). *Kafka: Toward a Minor Literature*. Minneapolis, MN: University of Minnesota Press.

Deleuze, G., and Guattari, F. (1994). *What is Philosophy?* London: Verso.

Deleuze, G., and Parnet, C. (1987). *Dialogues* (H. Tomlinson and B. Habberjam, Trans.). New York: Columbia University Press.

Dickens, C. (1952). *Our Mutual Friend. The Oxford Illustrated Dickens*. London: Oxford.

Drob, S. (2012). *Reading The Red Book: An Interpretive Guide to C. G. Jung's Liber Novus*. New Orleans: Spring.

Freud, S. (1925). The resistances to psycho-analysis. *The Standard Edition of the Complete Psychological Works of Sigmund Freud*, Vol. 19 (1923–1925), 211–24. London: Hogarth.

Freud, S. (1930). Civilization and its discontents. *The Standard Edition of the Complete Psychological Works of Sigmund Freud*, Vol. 21 (1927–1931), 64–145. London: Hogarth.

Gieser, S. (2014). Jung, Pauli, and the symbolic nature of reality. In H. Atmanspacher and C. Fuchs (Eds.), *The Pauli-Jung Conjecture and Its Impact Today*, 151–80. Exeter: Imprint Academic.

Henderson, D. (2014). *Apophatic Elements in the Theory and Practice of Psychoanalysis: Pseudo-Dionysius and C. G. Jung*. London: Routledge.

Hillman, J. (1964). *Suicide and the Soul*. New York: Harper & Row.

Hogenson, G. (2014). 'The wealth of the soul exists in images': From medieval icons to modern science. In T. Kirsch and G. Hogenson (Eds.), *The Red Book: Reflections on C. G. Jung's Liber Novus*, 94–107. London: Routledge.

Jenkins, B. (2016). *Eros and Economy: Jung, Deleuze, Sexual Difference*. London: Routledge.

Jung, C. G. (1956). *The Collected Works of C. G. Jung* (Sir H. Read, M. Fordham, and G. Adler, Eds.; W. McGuire, Exec. Ed.; R. F. C. Hull, Trans.) [hereafter *Collected Works*], Vol. 5, *Symbols of Transformation*. Princeton, NJ: Princeton University Press.

Jung, C. G. (1959a). Archetypes of the collective unconscious (1954). In *Collected Works*, Vol. 9i, *The Archetypes and the Collective Unconscious*, 3–41. New York: Pantheon.

Jung, C. G. (1959b). The psychology of the child archetype (1941). In *Collected Works*, Vol. 9i, *Archetypes of the Collective Unconscious*, 149–81. New York: Pantheon.

Jung, C. G. (1959c). *Collected Works*, Vol. 9ii, *Aion: Researches into the Phenomenology of the Self*. Princeton, NJ: Princeton University Press.

Jung, C. G. (1964). The meaning of psychology for modern man (1933). In *Collected Works*, Vol. 10, *Civilization in Transition*, 134–56. Princeton, NJ: Princeton University Press.

Jung, C. G. (1966). On the relation of analytical psychology to poetry (1922). In *Collected Works*, Vol. 15, *The Spirit in Man, Art, and Literature*, 65–83. New York: Pantheon.

Jung, C. G. (1989). *Memories, Dreams, Reflections*. New York: Vintage Books.

Jung, C. G. (1993a). Is there a Freudian type of poetry? (1932). In *Collected Works*, Vol. 18, *The Symbolic Life*, 765–66. London: Routledge.

Jung, C. G. (1993b). The Tavistock lectures (1935). In *Collected Works*, Vol. 18, *The Symbolic Life*, 3–182. London: Routledge.

Kaiser, B. M. (2017). Symptomatology. In M. Bunz, B. M. Kaiser, and K. Thiele (Eds.), *Symptoms of the Planetary Condition: A Critical Vocabulary*, 185–89. Lüneburg: meson press eG.

Kerslake, C. (2002). The vertigo of philosophy: Deleuze and the problem of immanence. *Radical Philosophy*, *113*: 10–23.

Kerslake, C. (2004). Rebirth through incest: On Deleuze's early Jungianism. *Angeliki: Journal of the Theoretical Humanities*, *9*(1):135–57.

Kerslake, C. (2006). Insects and incest: from Bergson and Jung to Deleuze. Accessed at www.multitudes.net/insects-and-incest-from-bergson/.

Kerslake, C. (2007). *Deleuze and the Unconscious*. London: Continuum.

Kerslake, C. (2009). Deleuze and the meanings of immanence. Accessed at http://after1968.org/app/webroot/uploads/Deleuze%20and%20the%20 Meanings%20of%20Immanence.doc.

Lovat, T., and Semetsky, I. (2009). Practical mysticism and Deleuze's ontology of the virtual. *Cosmos and History: The Journal of Natural and Social Philosophy 5*(2): 236–249.

McMillan, C. (2012). Archetypal intuition: Beyond the human. In D. Henderson (Ed.), *Psychoanalysis, Culture and Society*, 38–66. Newcastle: Cambridge Scholars Publishing.

McMillan, C. (2018). Jung and Deleuze: enchanted openings to the Other: A philosophical contribution. *International Journal of Jungian Studies*, *10*(3): 184–98.

Pannell, B. (2018). Deleuze's critical and clinical uses of literature. *Annual Review of Critical Psychology*, *14*: 193–209.

Rowland, S. (2005). *Jung as a Writer*. Hove: Routledge.

Sedgwick, D. (1993). *Jung and Searles*. London: Routledge.

Semetsky, I. (2004). The complexity of individuation. *International Journal of Applied Psychoanalytic Studies*, *1*(4): 324–46.

Semetsky, I. (2006). *Deleuze, Education and Becoming*. Rotterdam: Sense Publishers.

Semetsky, I., and Delpech-Ramey, J. (2012). Jung's psychology and Deleuze's philosophy: The unconscious in learning. *Educational Philosophy and Theory*, *44*(1): 69–81.

Smith, D. (1997). Introduction: 'A life of pure immanence': Deleuze's 'Critique et clinique' project. In G. Deleuze, *Essays Critical and Clinical*, xi–liii. Minneapolis, MN: University of Minnesota Press.

Stern, D. (1985). *The Interpersonal World of the Infant: A View from Psychoanalysis and Developmental Psychology*. New York: Basic.

Zeller, M. (1975). *The Dream: The Vision of the Night*. Sheridan, WY: Fisher King Press.

Žižek, S. (2004). Notes on a debate 'From within the people'. *Criticism*, *46*(4): 661–666.

Zourabichvili, F. (1996). Six notes on the percept (On the relation between the critical and the clinical). In P. Paton (Ed.), *Deleuze: A Critical Reader*, 188–216. Oxford: Blackwell.

Chapter 4

One, two, three... one

The edusemiotic self

Inna Semetsky

Individuation as becoming-self

Edusemiotics – educational semiotics – is a new field of study that explores semiotics as a foundational philosophy in the context of education and learning. Semiotics is the study of signs, their action and transformation. Signs are not just visible objects referring to something else directly. Jung seems to propagate this fallacy: he took symbols as standing for more than their immediate meanings, and signs as representing something already known (as penis, father or mother, for Freud). But, according to the founder of modern semiotics, American philosopher Charles S. Peirce, signs represent a broad category encompassing images, indices, and symbols as well as signs portending in nature. Signs also include clinical symptoms in terms of both diagnosis and prognosis. Signs are *relational* entities. Gilles Deleuze conceptualised 'fold' as an in-between relation. Jung commented that Freud 'was blind toward the paradox and ambiguity of the contents of the unconscious, and did not know that everything which arises out of the unconscious has [...] an inside and an outside' (Jung 1963: 153) – quite in accord with Deleuze for whom the 'outside' is

> animated by [...] movements, folds and foldings that [...] make up an inside: they are not something other than the outside but precisely the inside *of* the outside. [...] The inside is an operation of the outside: [...] an inside [...] is [...] the fold of the outside.
>
> (Deleuze 1988a: 96–97)

Deleuze considered philosophers and creative artists to be semioticians and symptomatologists who can *unfold* and read signs as symptoms. This attention to signs and images was prominent in Deleuze's overall corpus, and his philosophy partakes of the Hermetic hieroglyphic worldview that considered the world as a book written with signs to be deciphered. Deleuze and Guattari were strongly anti-Oedipal and their critique included both Freud's and Jung's (re)turn to the 'royal road' of dreams. Yet, Jung was explicit that:

> The *via regia* to the unconscious [...] is not the dream, as he [Freud] thought, but the complex, which is the architect of dreams and of symptoms. Nor is this *via* so very 'royal', either, since the way pointed out by the complex is more like a rough and uncommonly devious footpath that often loses itself in the undergrowth and generally leads not into the heart of the unconscious but past it.
>
> (CW 8: §210)

Complexes express deep psychic life, and the unconscious is not reduced to its repressed 'acquisitions' during an individual lifetime but has a collective dimension in terms of *objective* psyche. The collective unconscious is populated by archetypes that manifest in typical life-situations as habitual patterns of thought and action of which we remain unaware, therefore tending to behave repetitively, thus reinforcing the archetypal constellations that sink even deeper in the unconscious to the point of having totally possessed the psyche. Jung emphasised that 'complexes can *have us*' (CW 8: §200), and a feeling-toned complex is 'the *image* of a certain psychic situation [...]. This image has a powerful inner coherence, it has its own wholeness and [...] a relatively high degree of autonomy' (CW 8: §201). Complexes partake of 'Descartes' devils and seem to delight in playing impish tricks' (CW 8: §202) leading to the fragmentation of personality. They form splinter psyches or 'the fractured I of a dissolved Cogito' (Deleuze 1994: 194). For Jung, these fractured pieces are to be integrated within the psyche made whole. It is the archetype of wholeness – or self – that implicitly guides us towards 'the ultimate integration of conscious and unconscious, or [...] the assimilation of the ego to a wider personality' (CW 8: §557): the process of individuation.

In analysis, individuation as a healing (making whole) process was defined by Jung in terms of *self-education*: becoming an integrated personality, becoming-self. The *edusemiotic self* thus indicates individuation as a symbolic process of self-education and learning that proceeds by means of the integration of the unconscious guided by the archetype of wholeness, the self. Presenting his depth psychology as a method of self-education, Jung (CW 17) maintained that self-knowledge remains an indispensable basis of adult development and emphasised the indirect method for attaining such inner self-knowledge by means of symbolic mediation when we learn to 'perceive the effects [of the unconscious] that come into consciousness' (ibid.: §112). While being 'irrepresentable' (CW 8: §417) factors at the invisible end of the total psychic spectrum, archetypes are 'the forms which the instincts assume. [...] It is like Nature herself – prodigiously conservative, and yet transcending her own historical conditions in her acts of creation' (CW 8: §339). The archetypes thus function as signs subsisting in the world that, like hieroglyphs to be deciphered, *relate* to something that they are not, something *other* – therefore forming enfolded structures, the meaning of which is not given *a priori* but needs to be interpreted in practice. Jung refers to what he calls the Faustian question when 'the ego must [...] ask: "How am I affected by this sign?"' (CW 8: §188), that is, by one or another invisible archetype within the individuating process.

For Deleuze (1995: 127), the role of *affects* is significant: affects are 'becomings that spill over beyond whoever lives through them (thereby becoming someone else)'. Commenting on the case of Little Hans, Deleuze remarked that Freud took no account of the collective assemblages comprising multiple becomings as 'moving relationships' (Deleuze and Parnet 1987: 93) which constitute the process of individuation that demands we become aware of the imperceptible signs affecting us at the unconscious level. It is precisely a function of 'consciousness not only to recognize and assimilate the external world through the gateway of the senses, but to translate into visible reality the world within us' (CW 8: §342). Such making the invisible visible or perceiving the imperceptible constitutes a mystical experience, which Deleuze (1989) equated with a sudden awakening of perception that is raised to a new power. In Jungian analysis, such 'vision' is the index of wholeness achieved by means of the transcendent function – a term borrowed from the mathematics of complex (real and imaginary) numbers. The compensatory relation between the unconscious and consciousness, writes Jung:

> generates a tension charged with energy and creates a living, third thing – not a logical stillbirth in accordance with the principle *tertium non datur* but a movement out of the suspension between opposites, a living birth that leads to a new level of being, a new situation. The transcendent function manifests itself as a quality of conjoined opposites.
>
> (CW 8: §189)

Tertium non datur – the *excluded* third – pertains to pure rationality, the logic of the non-affective intellect. Jung's depth psychology aims to integrate the unconscious by the inclusion of 'a third thing in which the opposites can unite. [...] In nature the resolution of opposites is always an energic process: she acts *symbolically* in the truest sense of the word, doing something that expresses both sides, just as a waterfall visibly mediates between above and below' (CW 14: §705). The waterfall as 'the incommensurable third' (CW 14: §705) serves as a powerful symbol, a precursor for individuation that parallels Deleuze's concept of becoming, which always 'passes *between* points, it comes up through the middle. [...] A becoming is neither one nor two; [...] it is the in-between, the [...] line of flight or descent running perpendicular to both' (Deleuze and Guattari 1987: 293) – just like in Jung's ingenious example of the waterfall. The *tertium non datur* hence becomes *tertium quid* – the *included* third: even if apparently logically unclassifiable, it establishes a *relation* that connects the perceived opposites.

For Jung, 'archetypes [as] [...] structural elements of the psyche [...] possess a certain autonomy and specific energy which enables them to attract, out of the conscious mind, those contents which are best suited to themselves' (CW 5: §344) and are charged with psychic or spiritual energy, exceeding Freud's sexual libido. While Deleuze seems to think that not only Freud but Jung too reduced libido to an immediate satisfaction of one's wishes, he (with Guattari) inadvertently used the term *libido* in quite a Jungian manner, designating specific *energy* and the transformations of this energy in terms of the role of the unconscious as active *desiring-production* that overturns the theatre of static representations by laying down *the plane of immanence* or the plane of Nature: 'immanence is the unconscious itself' (Deleuze 1988b: 29). Significantly, Deleuze does not deny the presence of the 'transcendental principle [that] *precedes* matter and form, species and parts, and every other element of the constituted individual' (Deleuze 1994: 38) while acting at an invisible plane of organisation:

> It is like in music where the principle of composition is not given in a directly perceptible, audible, relation with what it provides. It is therefore a plane of transcendence, a kind of design, in the mind of man or in the mind of a god, even when it is accorded a maximum of immanence by plunging it into the depth of Nature, or of the Unconscious.
>
> (Deleuze and Parnet 1987: 91)

The aim of schizoanalysis – coined by Deleuze and Guattari (1983) to contrast with psychoanalysis – is to rediscover the transcendental unconscious defined by the immanence of its criteria and to articulate the corresponding practice which is hereto qualified as *both* transcendental *and* materialist, '*an unconscious of thought* just as profound as *the unknown of the body*' (Deleuze 1988b: 19). Such status of the unconscious indicates a convergence between Deleuze's and Jung's positions, and especially in terms of the complementary relation between as-if-irreconcilable dualities. Jung considered the real nature of the archetypes to be transcendental and occupying what he called the unitary or *psychoid* level, which reflects the 'secret immanence of the divine spirit of life' (CW 14: §623) partaking of the alchemical *benedicta viriditas* or 'blessed green' as a sign of the presence of the animating power in matter that creates one world: *unus mundus*. The archetypal dynamics are 'a manifestation of the energy that springs from the tension of opposites' (CW 7: §121), and it is when the conscious ego acknowledges the existence of an unconscious partner that such semiotic communication puts one on the road to individuation in order 'to free life from where it's trapped' (Deleuze 1995: 141).

Even if Jung made clear that the 'solvent' to the problem of unification 'can only be of an irrational nature' (CW 14: §705), there is a specific, even if paradoxical, logic that underlies the Western esoteric tradition of Hermeticism, Kabbalah and alchemy. This is what

Deleuze calls the logic of multiplicities and which is at the crux of edusemiotics.

Logic of multiplicities

According to Jung, alchemy purports to fill in the gaps in religious dogma, which demonstrates a tendency towards the masculine, with the opposite, compensatory tendency of invoking 'the chthonic femininity of the unconscious' (CW 12: §26). Across his corpus, Jung referred to the axiom of Maria Prophetissa, a third-century alchemist, as a metaphor for individuation. The enigmatic axiom states: *One becomes two, two becomes three, and out of the third comes the one as the fourth.* Jung's interpretation of the axiom boils down to his *quaternity* as the unity of the four elements, even if one of them appears missing – like an inferior function marking the deficiency in consciousness. But Jung seems to take the sequence of numbers literally, in their linear progression. From the viewpoint of edusemiotics, though, these numbers symbolise what Deleuze referred to as *multiplicities* that possess a specific logic in contrast to binary logic, the latter utilising the principle of the excluded middle as *tertium non datur.* In parallel to Charles S. Peirce's notion of genuine signs as triadic structures, Deleuze points out that 'there are two in the second, to the point where there is a firstness in the secondness, and there are three in the third' (Deleuze 1989: 30). Multiplicities are intensive, interpenetrative: they are ternary structures functioning on the basis of 'a theory and practice of relations, of the AND' (Deleuze and Parnet 1987: 15) that form assemblages as systems of signs based on 'symbiosis, a "sympathy"' (ibid.: 69). Multiplicity's 'only unity is that of co-functioning' (ibid.: 69) – of sympathetic relations forming a complex whole. Such logic is not 'subordinate to the verb to be. [...] Substitute the AND for IS. A *and* B. The AND is [...] the path of all relations, which makes relations shoot outside their terms' (ibid.: 57).

Taking two abstract terms A and B, Deleuze inserts the conjunction AND that defies the opposition between the binaries. A multiplicity contains an a-signifying rupture or *difference* – a pure relation, a gap – in which the conjunction AND intervenes in the mode of the included third: not in the opposition of A to B but 'in their complementarity'

...AND

...AND

AND

Figure 4.1 Multiplicity

(Deleuze and Parnet 1987: 131). Even as A and B formally belong to different, heterogeneous series, they reciprocally determine each other. 'It is in difference that movement is produced as an "effect", that phenomena flash their meaning like signs', notes Deleuze (1994: 57). Recall Jung's example of the waterfall in nature as an 'effect' or the included middle that resolves the perceived opposition. Deleuze ingeniously addresses difference in primarily ontological terms: 'Difference is not phenomenon but the noumenon closest to the phenomenon. [...] The phenomenon that flashes across this system, bringing about the communication between disparate series, is a sign' (ibid.: 222). Such communication is *transversal*, assuring the mutual 'affectivity' or resonance of A and B. Deleuze intensifies AND as if stuttering: AND... AND... AND, and we can construct a visual diagram for multiplicity as a semiotic structure where the otherwise divergent series symbolised by two 'disparates', A and B, converge on a paradoxical element symbolised by AND (Figure 4.1).

The included third creates a rhizomatic network in which the whole dualistic split of *either* sensible *or* intelligible, *either* rational thought *or* lived experience, *either* material *or* spiritual, is bridged. Rhizome is Deleuze's biological metaphor for becoming, a living symbol of vitality and organic growth. Jung would agree:

> Life has always seemed to me like a plant that lives on its rhizome. Its true life is invisible, hidden in the rhizome. The part that appears above ground lasts only a single summer. Then it withers away – an ephemeral apparition. [...] Yet I have never lost a sense

of something that lives and endures underneath the eternal flux. What we see is the blossom, which passes. The rhizome remains.

(Jung 1963: 4)

Such a hidden, invisible, *true life* is 'a' life of pure immanence (Deleuze 2001). Deleuze uses the indefinite article – 'a' life – as an index or a sign of the *impersonal* transcendental field, which is 'a-subjective' (2001: 25) – outside individual consciousness – hence unconscious in the Jungian sense. Immanence and transcendence are not simple binary opposites but are enfolded, with 'the immanent contained within a transcendental field' (Deleuze 2001: 30). They are just two poles in the single, ubiquitous semiotic relation.

Jung refers to the Hermetic principle of *coincidentia oppositorum* as 'transgressivity' (CW 8: §964), the mystical coincidence of opposites, such as matter and spirit, that nonetheless can be connected indirectly or transversally via the semiotic conjunction AND. Deleuze describes transversal communication in almost alchemical terms as the 'transformation of substances and a dissolution of forms, a passage to the limit or flight from contours [...]. We witness the incorporeal power of that intense matter, the material power of that language' (Deleuze and Guattari 1987: 109) expressed in symbolic form. It is via symbols and images that we become aware of the unconscious knowledge as gnosis. A symbolic approach 'reflects a higher level of intellect and, by not forcibly representing the unknowable as known, gives a more faithful picture of the real state of affairs' (CW 11: §417). Gnosis is produced in the midst of the transformative process (semiosis) that connects two 'inseparable planes in reciprocal presupposition' (Deleuze and Guattari 1987: 109) via their integration, and 'establish[es] the bond of a profound complicity between nature and mind' (Deleuze 1994: 165) that manifests at the deeper, soul, level – the soul of the world, *anima mundi*.

Deleuze brings in Hermetic notions, referring to the transversal link as a demonic operation that leaps over borders and boundaries. Significantly, it is Diotima the Priestess – a feminine figure – who taught Socrates that there is a 'daimon' by the name of Eros located between 'lack' and 'plenty' that can hold two opposites together as a whole. As a culmination of desire sparked between the two deities, Eros itself is a symbol of union (alchemical marriage), of *hieros gamos* or *coniunctio*

(CW 8: §900). It is the erotic desire for gnosis, or longing for wisdom, that ultimately brings the unconscious into consciousness. For Jung, Eros is the feminine principle of relatedness, of binding, of connecting, in contrast to detached reason or Logos (e.g., CW 9ii: §29). In Jung's dreams, the figure of Philemon, his male spiritual guide, was accompanied by a female figure as a personification of soul. Jung shared the Gnostic vision of Wisdom-Sophia as the Bride of Christ who, by educating humankind in gnosis, can bring Sophia back into Pleroma (fullness of being). Jung associated Wisdom with one of the Sephirot in the Kabbalistic Tree of Life, which is a symbol of the divine descending into the human world. Deleuze, non-incidentally, asserted that *becoming-woman* is 'the key to all other becomings' (Deleuze and Guattari 1987: 277). Sophia resides in all of us, even the most phallocratic, as remnants of divine sparks enfolded in the world that need to be gathered, unconcealed, or unfolded so as to create a life 'filled with immanence' (Deleuze 1997: 137).

Eros, affect, desire, libido! Whatever the name, it cannot be reduced to merely the lack posited by psychoanalysis: it is the excess (or 'plenty') of implicated, enfolded meanings that characterises schizoanalytic desiring-production as the individuating process of becoming-other, becoming-self. Desire is *'constructivist'* (Deleuze and Parnet 1987: 96): it constructs the plane of immanence. Eros, according to myth, was conceived in an uncanny act that partakes of Deleuze's description of the plane of immanence:

> it implies a sort of groping experimentation and its layout resorts to measures that are not very respectable, rational, or reasonable. These measures belong to the order of dreams, of pathological processes, esoteric experiences, drunkenness, and excess. We head for the horizon, on the plane of immanence, and we return with bloodshot eyes, yet they are the eyes of the mind.
>
> (Deleuze and Guattari 1994: 41)

It is the eyes of the mind that allow us to perceive the invisible archetypes of the collective unconscious when, by constructing the plane of immanence, we can cross the threshold of consciousness. Such an erotic, active relation pertains to the paradoxical logic of multiplicities (signs) and showcases itself in *synchronistic*, a-causal experiences defying the direct mechanistic causality of classical physics. The concept of synchronicity was developed by Jung in collaboration with physicist and Nobel-laureate Wolfgang Pauli. Synchronicity addresses the problematic of the meaningful 'relation of the psychic to the material world [that can be compared] with two cones, whose apices, meeting in a point without extension – a real zero-point – touch and do not touch' (CW 8: §418), just like the intensive yet seemingly 'non-localizable' (Deleuze 1994: 83) conjunction AND that forms a semiotic triangle as a paradoxical open-enclosure. Albeit virtual, such a point would not be 'without similarities to the One-Whole of the Platonists' (Deleuze 1991: 93). Pauli envisaged the development of theories of the unconscious as outgrowing their solely therapeutic applications by being eventually assimilated into mainstream natural science. He considered the unconscious analogous to the notion of '"field" in physics' (Pauli 1994: 164). Indeed, 'the unconscious belongs to the realm of physics' (Deleuze and Guattari 1983: 283), to complex nature that exceeds the physical reality given directly to the senses. Reality is semiotic, permeated with signs that can reach deep into the unconscious virtual memories. The 'virtual is the whole' (Deleuze 2003a: 30), and the field of the collective unconscious constitutes a cosmic, collective 'gigantic memory' (Deleuze 2001: 212) contained in the transcendental field.

So, when Maria Prophetissa 'cried without restraint, "One becomes two, two becomes three, and out of the third comes the One as the fourth"' (as Jung says in *Psychology and Alchemy* [CW 12: §209], quoting from the alchemical text) – likely similar to Cassandra in her frenzy crying out, in vain, about the future destruction of Troy – she was using these numbers *symbolically*. Sure enough, the mode of expression pertaining to multiplicities is 'a virtual number' (Deleuze 2003a: 34). Deleuze stresses, in reference to Peirce, that there is 'not merely 1, 2, 3, but 1, 2 in 2 and 1, 2, 3 in 3' (Deleuze 1986: 198) – even if he erroneously thinks that Peirce meant thirdness as the end of the story (that as such would have *closed* a semiotic triangle). But it is precisely thirdness (*tertium quid*) that is the very *essence* of the unending semiotic process, the evolutionary dynamics of signs: 'Essence is finally the third term that [...] complicates the sign and the meaning. [...] It measures in each case their relation [...] the degree of their unity' (Deleuze 2000: 90), and it is the very 'essence of the virtual to be actualized' (Deleuze 2003a: 28). It is because of the relational, semiotic structure of the world that 'From virtuals we descend to actual states of affairs, and from states of affairs we ascend to virtuals, without being able to isolate one from the other' (Deleuze and Guattari 1994: 160).

The ultimate inseparability or unity of the 'one world' manifests in synchronistic experiences. Synchronicity demonstrates that 'psyche and matter are two different aspects of one and the same thing' (CW 8: §418). This thing is *meaning* as the included third, the conjunction AND – a *paradoxical yet logical* element in the ubiquitous tri-relative semiotic structure. So 'one' as becoming 'two' means duality – the opposition of matter and mind, consciousness and the unconscious at the level of our ordinary, sensible experience. But 'two' duly becomes 'three' in their reconciliation: the alchemical 'union of the two is a kind of self-fertilization' (CW 12: §209). There is no place in the one-sided logic of consciousness for such apparent self-reference or self-organisation, precisely because of the latter's circularity or nonlinearity. It is when a semiotic triangle is 'complete' by virtue of conjunction that it simultaneously becomes another 'one' as the 'fourth' in the continuous transformation of signs or, in Bergson's terms, creative evolution. Signs evolve: they grow in meaning. The growth of meanings *per se* is a mark of 'infinite "learning"' (Deleuze 1994: 192): novelty is the prerogative of the evolution of consciousness and is the ultimate task of edusemiotics because 'Everything that teaches us something emits signs; every act of learning is an interpretation of signs' (Deleuze 2000: 4). The semiotic structure of multiplicities highlights the repetition of difference and not the reproduction of sameness.

Strictly speaking, the fourth is 'one' in terms of the *integrated whole*, a sort of 'area' of the semiotic triangle. In Jungian analysis, the integration of the unconscious 'presents a way of moving from "either-or" to "and" by going beyond the limitations of logical discourse or common sense. [...] The experience of "and-ness" is central to psychological change' (Samuels 1985: 59). Surely Deleuze's conjunction AND cannot be reduced to simple numerical addition. Deleuze presents the logic of multiplicities in terms of the esoteric calculus of Ideas, which are obscure problematic instances that, just like signs, are 'differential flashes which leap and metamorphose' (Deleuze 1994: 146). They are not *a priori* clear and distinct, as Descartes wanted them to be. They are unconscious structures 'necessarily overlaid by their products or effects' (Deleuze 2003a: 181) that, like Jungian archetypes, can jolt us out of the comfort zone of habits, thus forcing the 'genesis of the act of thought' (Deleuze 1994: 157). The Ideas comprise 'a theatre of problems and always open questions which draws spectator, setting and characters into the real movement of an apprenticeship of the entire unconscious, the final elements of which remain the problems themselves' (Deleuze 1994: 192). Indeed, the field of collective unconscious can never be fully exhausted because of the archetypes' manifold of references.

Jung's self-education as an *apprenticeship in signs* necessarily becomes an 'experimentation on oneself, [which] is our only identity, our single chance for all the combinations which inhabit us' (Deleuze and Parnet 1987: 11). It is problematic Ideas that elicit learning by virtue of the 'presentation of the unconscious, not the representation of consciousness' (Deleuze 1994: 192). Learning from the experiential, albeit perplexing, encounters with archetypes ultimately creates the 'widened consciousness' which:

> is no longer that touchy egotistical bundle of personal wishes, fears, hopes and ambitions which always has to be compensated or corrected by unconscious counter-tendencies; instead it is a function of relationship to the world of objects, bringing the individual into absolute, binding, and indissoluble communion with the world at large.
>
> (CW 7: §275)

Deleuze's powerful method that enables the integration of unconscious Ideas is both empirical and transcendental. The *both-and* quality is intrinsic to semiotics. Recall the *psychoid*, or psychophysical, status of the archetypal – semiotic – reality. While maintaining the dictum of empiricism in terms of relations being external to their terms, signs as differential relations or pure *differences* do determine these very terms, thus being their constitutive – transcendental – condition ('one becomes two...' etc.). Transcendental empiricism is superior to its plain *tabula-rasa* cousin. Jung too denounced the *tabula-rasa* state of individual consciousness because the 'collective unconscious comprises in itself the psychic life of our ancestors right back to the earliest beginnings. It is the matrix of all conscious psychic occurrences' (CW 8: §230). The world is populated by problematic Ideas, which are virtual; yet it is on the basis of the very *reality* of the virtual 'that existence is produced, in accordance with a time and a space immanent in the Idea' (Deleuze 1994: 211) when we experience the effects of actualised archetypes. Their integration in consciousness demands a reciprocal *counter-actualisation*: moving, via mediation by symbols, from the actual back to the virtual.

A semiotic relation has 'two halves of the Symbol' (Deleuze 1994: 279), and signs always participate in the double, Neo-platonic, movement of descending and ascending while effectuating 'the genesis of intuition in intelligence' (Deleuze 1991: 111). Intuition blended with intelligence is the way of reading signs, of exploring and evaluating the problematic Ideas. The encountered 'problem is at once both transcendent and immanent in relation to its solutions. Transcendent, because it consists in a system of ideal liaisons or differential relations between genetic elements. Immanent, because these liaisons or relations are incarnated in the actual relations which do not resemble them and are defined by the field of solution' (Deleuze 1994: 163). It is the *incarnation* or *embodiment* of the transcendental field of the collective unconscious that allows it to merge with its own 'object' as deep knowledge, gnosis, which is always already immanent in perception even if in its vague, virtual, albeit not in any way unknowable, Kantian, state. The Idea's 'problematic structure is part of objects themselves, allowing them to be grasped as signs, just as the questioning or problematising instance is a part of knowledge allowing its positivity and its specificity to be grasped in the act of *learning*' (Deleuze 1994: 64).

The logic of multiplicities, of signs, thus literally *makes sense*: meaning is implicated in learning! There is no genuine learning in what can be immediately recognised: objects directly given to consciousness are only surface effects, the pale projections or derivatives of the 'initially undifferentiated field' (Deleuze 1993: 10) of the collective unconscious. Yet it is precisely a surface – serving as a symbolic border between material and spiritual, corporeal and incorporeal – that functions as the 'locus of *sense:* signs remain deprived of sense as long as they do not enter into the surface organization which assures the resonance of two series' (Deleuze 1990: 104). Archetypal experiences begin to make sense (thereby initiating individuation) when the depth of the psyche 'having been spread out became width. The becoming unlimited is maintained entirely within this inverted width' (Deleuze 1990: 9), and the meaning of experience, paradoxically, even 'more profound since *it* occurs at the surface' (Deleuze 1990: 10) in the form of projection of deep unconscious structures. The logic of multiplicities transcends the one-sided 'syntactical link with a world' (Deleuze 1990: 178). It has its own grammar. The impoverished link is transformed into a synchronistic or transversal connection that includes the dimension of meaning and makes logic commensurate with ethics.

The ethics of integration

Deleuze addresses the paradoxes of logic mainly in relation to language, but the French word *sens* – or meaning – also has an ethical nuance in terms of the direction taken in our practical lives. The meaning produced in experience affects our decision-making and choice of action, and we always have 'to become worthy of the event' (Deleuze and Guattari 1994: 160). The diversity of experiential situations that abound in life disrupts preconceived judgements based on a strict moral code, especially when problematic situations present us with moral dilemmas. Morality cannot be imposed as though 'brought down on tables of stone from Sinai' (CW 7: §30), and the presupposed universal rules of human conduct can 'never lead to those crucial decisions which are the turning-points in a man's life. […] Through the new ethic, the ego-consciousness is ousted from its central position in a psyche organized on the lines of a monarchy or totalitarian state, its place being taken by *wholeness* or the *self*, which is now recognized as central' (Jung in Neumann 1969: 13, 18). The new ethics is holistic, devoted to the integration of the unconscious shadow, in contrast to the old or partial ethics focused solely on ego-consciousness. Archetypes can be 'the ruling powers' (CW 7: §151), and amidst the archetypes such as anima and animus, great mother, eternal child, trickster, old wise man, rebirth, persona, etc., the shadow can easily affect the psyche to the point of possession. One's own shadowy, unsavoury qualities tend to become projected onto the other. At the collective level, the shadow encompasses those outside the norms of the established moral or legal order and social system, such as 'criminals, psychotics, misfits, scapegoats' (Samuels 1985: 66). It is not only that these figures belong to the category of outsiders – significantly, it is dominant culture itself that fails to assimilate its own shadow and as a result often implements the scapegoat policy because of its reliance on 'universality, method [...] judgement [...] a court of reason, a pure 'right' of thought. [...] The exercise of thought thus conforms to [...] the dominant meanings and to the requirements of the established order' (Deleuze and Parnet 1987: 13).

Even as ego-consciousness focuses on indubitable and unequivocal moral principles, these very principles crumble under the '*compensatory significance of the shadow* in the light of ethical responsibility' (Jung in Neumann 1969: 12), the neglect of which tends to precipitate multiple consequences in the social world. The shadow rules one-sidedly unless integrated into the whole of the personality. In the absence of integration, it can create a sealed, aggressive world until it starts spontaneously acting out, often in the form of a destructive climax or psychotic breakdown. Individuation as becoming-self is embedded in the dynamics of becoming-other, and it is the confrontation with the shadow that brings to the surface the conscious 'recognition of an alien "other" in oneself' (CW 13: §481). Deleuze commented that culture usually experiences violence that serves as an active force for the formation of our thinking: force is 'an act of the fold' (Deleuze 1993: 18) in the individuating process that includes 'the harshest exercise in depersonalization' (Deleuze 1995: 6) as a dark precursor for becoming-other, becoming-self! Yet, without undergoing a symbolic death, no rebirth is possible. It is affective becoming-other that 'draws a hidden universe out of the shadow' (Deleuze and Guattari 1994: 66), illuminating it like a beam of light so that a tiny 'spark can flash [...] to make us see and think what was lying in the shadow around the words, things we were hardly aware existed' (Deleuze 1995: 141). A spark, as a counterpart to the shadow, may very well belong to the divine sparks of Kabbalistic vessels dispersed in the world, the integration of which parallels the archetype of rebirth that Jung equated with the affirmation of life. Rebirth is characterised by our lives acquiring novel sense and direction in the process of unfolding the archetypal structures that 'imply ways of living, possibilities of existence, they're the symptoms of life gushing forth or draining away. [...] There's a profound link between signs, events, life and vitalism' (Deleuze 1995: 143).

The value dimension is inherent in the interpretation of signs, and the process of becoming is 'ethical and aesthetic, as opposed to morality' (ibid.: 114). We trace the multiple rhizomatic lines by going to the depth of the problem: 'which of them are dead-ended or blocked, which cross voids, which continue, and most importantly the line of steepest gradient, how it draws in the rest, towards what destination' (Deleuze and Parnet 1987: 120). The immanent evaluation of experience brings forth the *clinical* aspect of Deleuze's philosophy not only by entailing a *diagnosis* of a particular mode of existence by means of assessing its symptoms – that is, reading them as the signs of the present. It also affords a *prognosis* even if uncertain. Deleuze asks, prophetically, 'What is it which tells us that, on a line of flight, we will not rediscover everything we were fleeing? […] How can one avoid the line of flight's becoming identical with a pure and simple movement of self-destruction' (Deleuze and Parnet 1987: 38). The clinical aspect is complemented by *critical* and *creative* aspects, and:

> The problem of critique is that of the value of values, of the evaluation from which their value arises, thus the problem of their *creation*. […] This is the crucial point; *high* and *low, noble* and *base*, are not values but represent the differential element from which the value of values themselves derives.
>
> (Deleuze 1983: 1–2)

Once again we are reminded that signs as multiplicities do not involve 'a simple addition' (Deleuze and Guattari 1987: 313): it is the *evaluation* of experience, the interpretation of signs, and getting to the *depth* of the differential dynamics that brings to the surface specific meanings enfolded in the psyche. A singular event 'upsets being' (Deleuze 1995: 44) while simultaneously propelling us to becoming, to individuation. Jung was explicit that the process of individuation, contrary to extreme individualism, produces 'a consciousness of human community precisely because it makes us aware of the unconscious, which unites and is common to all mankind' (CW 16: §227). By integrating the unconscious, we have a chance to become worthy of events and experiences as the creed of Deleuze's ethics.

The integration of the shadow thus becomes a specific method of ethics that may put an end to the continuing debate: 'since Socrates […] [philosophers] have sought […] criteria for distinguishing between right and wrong and between good and evil' (Baron, Pettit, and Slote 1997: 1). What is common to all approaches is that they are framed by the reasoning of a rational agent who presents moral categories in the form of binary opposites. The ethics of integration, however, overcomes the split inherent in simple moral algebra with its division into good versus evil or right versus wrong. It enables us to move beyond good and evil via the integration of those dualisms that are deeply ingrained in the cultural consciousness. The ethics of integration, the ultimate task of which is 'the design of an *open* society, a society of creators' (Deleuze 1991: 111), recapitulates the ontology of relations and focuses on new modes of existence, on multiple becomings. Becoming, for Deleuze, is an anti-memory or rather a paradoxical memory of the future, as if 'everything culminates in a "has been"'' (Deleuze 1990: 159), which is understandable, considering that signs are always bipolar, double-sided entities connecting the dimensions of past and future as two poles of one 'temporal' sign. A society of creators would comprise *a people to come* as the uncanny product of multiple experimentations. These people belong to 'an oppressed, bastard, lower, anarchical, nomadic, irremediably minor race. [...] They have resistance in common – their resistance to death, to servitude, to the intolerable, to shame, and to the present' (Deleuze and Guattari 1994: 109–10). Resistance to the present demands its evaluation, laying down the plane of immanence, reading signs, and 'decoding the secrets of intelligent alien life within and without us' (Ansell-Pearson 1997: 4). Such life is *neutral*, beyond the dualities of subject and object, self and other, good and evil, and the people to come will have to become edusemioticians, fluent in the language of signs and capable of applying it at the level of practice.

Coincidentally, Pauli envisaged the gradual discovery of a *neutral* language (in Meier 2001) that functions symbolically to describe an invisible reality which is inferable indirectly through its visible effects. Responding to Pauli, Jung pointed out the 'materialization of a potentially available reality, an actualization of the *mundus potentialis*' (in Meier, 2001: 83). Such language partakes of Deleuze's esoteric differential calculus, which is 'beyond good and evil' (Deleuze 1994: 182) as the prerogative of the *mathesis universalis*. Mathesis – also translated as *learning* – unifies science, art, spirituality and magic and represents 'an alphabet of what it means to think' (Deleuze 1994: 182). Deleuze is adamant that 'to believe that mathesis is merely a mystical lore, inaccessible and superhuman, would be a complete mistake.

[...] For mathesis deploys itself at the level of life, of living man. [...] Essentially, mathesis would be the exact description of human nature' (Deleuze 2007: 143) expressing itself in characters representing 'the *encounter* of the sensible object and the object of thought. The sensible object is called symbol, and the object of thought [...] is a hieroglyph or a cipher. [...] mathesis [...] transforms knowledge itself into a sensible object. Thus we shall see mathesis insist upon the correspondences between material and spiritual creation' (Deleuze 2007: 151) in the best tradition of Hermeticism. Such universal language transcends the barriers between native languages, conflicting beliefs, and incommensurable values immortalised in the symbol of 'the heaven-high tower of Babel that brought confusion to mankind' (CW 5: §171). Mathesis as a *neutral* language reflects the unified, psychoid reality of archetypes, and its 'real characters' are archetypal images, ideograms, or what Leibniz called 'arcana'.

From analysis to synthesis

Mathesis precedes and exceeds the verbal expressions of the conscious mind, and 'it is not the personal human being who is making the statement, but the archetype speaking through him' (Jung 1963: 352). Our knowledge of the language of images becomes of paramount importance because the process of individuation 'is an experience *in images and of images*. [...] Its beginning is almost invariably characterized by one's getting stuck in a blind alley or in some impossible situation; and its goal is [...] illumination or higher consciousness, by means of which the initial situation is overcome' (CW 9i: §82). It is via the archetypal images that the often-shocking encounter with the unconscious shadow in analysis is produced: 'the shock has an effect on the spirit, it forces it to think, and to think the Whole. [...] It does not follow like a logical effect, analytically, but synthetically as the dynamic effect of images [...] it is not a sum, but a "product", a unity of a higher order' (Deleuze 1989: 157–58) as the very purpose of individuation. While addressing in detail such esoteric practices as alchemy or *I Ching*, Jung also referred to 'the set of pictures in the Tarot cards [...] distantly descended from the archetypes of transformation' (CW 9i: §81) that represent 'typical situations, places, ways and means' (ibid.: §80) and not only active personalities in dreams.

The Tarot deck comprises 78 pictures, 22 so-called Major Arcana and 56 Minor. Deleuze, non-incidentally, says: 'I undo the folds of consciousness that pass through every one of my thresholds, the "twenty-two folds" that surround me and separate me from the deep' (Deleuze 1993: 93). Tarot performs a transcendent function in the form of a spatio-temporal, seemingly random, distribution of images in a typical layout (Semetsky 2011, 2013) as a Deleuzian 'dramatisation' of the virtual Ideas undergoing actualisation. There is 'drama beneath every logos' (Deleuze 2003a: 103) as the play of unconscious archetypes beneath their conceptual representation, the path to which is a transversal, synchronistic connection created in practice by an intuitive and 'unconscious psychic mechanism that engenders the perceived in consciousness' (Deleuze 1993: 95). A Tarot spread confirms 'the possibility and necessity of flattening all of the multiplicities on a single plane of consistency or exteriority' (Deleuze and Guattari 1987: 9) – the plane or *surface* on which we literally *see* the otherwise *invisible* elements of the psyche. The archetypal images 'convey the projection, on external space, of internal spaces defined by "hidden parameters" and variables or singularities of potential' (Deleuze 1993: 16). Still, hidden variables become exposed in our very experience: what was buried in the depth of the psyche is brought to the surface and the unconscious is made available to consciousness: it *makes sense.* Reading and interpreting the archetypal images of Tarot contributes to the integration of the unconscious in the process of counter-actualisation, as we said earlier: moving from the actual to the virtual so as to discover deep inner gnosis. Laying out the pictures creates a map or *cartography of the unconscious* that often suggests 'highs' or bouts of depression at the subtle, affective level. Tarot operates so as to 'bring this assemblage of the unconscious to the light of day, to select the whispering voices, to gather the tribes and secret idioms from which I extract something I call my Self' (Deleuze and Guattari 1987: 84): the individuated, edusemiotic self.

The interpretation of Tarot images parallels Jungian self-education in terms of symbolic lessons learned in the school of life that embody the meanings of experience, even as they so far remained out of awareness. Importantly, the Tarot 'map does not reproduce an unconscious closed in upon itself; it constructs the unconscious' (Deleuze and Guattari 1987: 12) in a process at once creative (making sense), critical

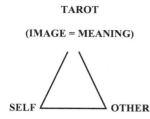

Figure 4.2 Tarot as a sign-system

(self-reflective), and clinical (healing). Tarot is a semiotic system *par excellence*, an exemplar of mathesis in action as the embodiment of the logic of the included third. It acts as the conjunction AND between consciousness and the unconscious, immanent and transcendent, self and other (Figure 4.2).

Jung stressed (CW 8: §402) that meaning and image are identical: as images unfold and take shape, their meanings become clear. Tarot images distributed in the layout comprise the semiotic 'levels of sensation […] like arrests or snapshots of motion, which […] recompose the movement synthetically in all its continuity' (Deleuze 2003b: 35). The edusemiotics of Tarot performs 'the supreme act of philosophy: not so much to think *THE* plane of immanence as to show that it is there, […] as the outside and inside of thought, […] that which cannot be thought and yet must be thought, which was thought once, as Christ was incarnated once, in order to show, that one time, the possibility of the impossible' (Deleuze and Guattari 1994: 59–60). Well, maybe not just that one time! It is the dynamic unfolding of signs that overcomes the dualism of the inside and the outside, consciousness and the unconscious, virtual and actual, and brings 'nature and culture together in its net' (Deleuze and Guattari 1987: 236). The relational nature–culture network is the precondition for the gnostic knowledge preeminent in spiritual teachings with regard to essential kinship and oneness with the world: mystics, creative artists, or 'supreme' philosophers play an intensive, participatory role in the world instead of remaining detached self-conscious observers.

The Tarot layout transcends 'spatial locations and temporal successions' (Deleuze 1994: 83) when the diachronic (historical, *ex-Memoria*) dimension of the collective unconscious becomes compactified into a single synchronic slice. We thus achieve an expanded perception of time and space when they are 'released from their human coordinates' (Deleuze 1986: 122). In this respect, 'Space-time ceases to be a pure given in order to become the totality or the nexus of differential relations in the subject, and the object itself ceases to be an empirical given in order to become the product of these relations' (Deleuze 1993: 89) – such *product* being the very *meaning* of experience embodied in the archetypal imagery of Tarot that 'determines the nature of the configurational process and the course it will follow, with seeming foreknowledge' (CW 8: §411), which differs from vulgar fortune telling but affords divinatory potential to Tarot readings!

Physicist David Bohm, whose ontology of wholeness is based on the existence of the implicate order of reality, asserted that there exists 'an anticipation of the future in the implicate order in the present. As they used to say, coming events cast their shadows in the present. Their shadows are being cast deep in the implicate order' (Bohm in Hederman 2003: 44). It is becoming aware of the archetypal shadow during Tarot readings that duly 'propels us into a hitherto unknown and unheard-of world of problems' (Deleuze 1994: 192). We are learning how to '*read*, find, retrieve the [semiotic] structures' (Deleuze 2003a: 181) in the form of material artefacts that embody our past, present, and even future experiences. By going deeper into the psyche we can explore options in the future evolution of signs and find a singular line of flight that 'has always been there, although it is the opposite of a destiny' (Deleuze and Parnet 1987: 125). Signs are *paradoxical* bipolar entities: the folds blending destiny with its own opposite, free will. Tarot creates '*an affect of self on self*' (Deleuze 1988a: 101) – and self-reference, because of the synthesis afforded by the logic of multiplicities, is simultaneously *self-transcendence*: individuation as becoming-self is always already becoming-other.

References

Ansell-Pearson, K. (1997). Deleuze outside/outside Deleuze. In K. Ansell-Pearson (Ed.), *Deleuze and Philosophy: The Difference Engineer* (pp. 1–22). London: Routledge.

Baron, M. W., Pettit, P., and Slote, M. (1997). *Three Methods of Ethics: A Debate*. Oxford: Wiley-Blackwell.

Deleuze, G. (1983). *Nietzsche and Philosophy* (H. Tomlinson, Trans.). New York: Columbia University Press.

Deleuze, G. (1986). *Cinema 1: The Movement-Image* (H. Tomlinson and B. Habberjam, Trans.). Minneapolis, MN: University of Minnesota.

Deleuze, G. (1988a). *Foucault* (S. Hand, Trans.). Minneapolis, MN: University of Minnesota Press.

Deleuze, G. (1988b). *Spinoza: Practical Philosophy* (R. Hurley, Trans.). San Francisco: City Lights Books.

Deleuze, G. (1989). *Cinema 2: The Time-Image* (H. Tomlinson and R. Galeta, Trans.). Minneapolis, MN: University of Minnesota.

Deleuze, G. (1990). *The Logic of Sense* (M. Lester and C. J. Stivale, Trans.). New York: Columbia University Press.

Deleuze, G. (1991). *Bergsonism* (H. Tomlinson, Trans.). New York: Zone Books.

Deleuze, G. (1993). *The Fold: Leibniz and the Baroque* (T. Conley, Trans.). Minneapolis, MN: University of Minnesota Press.

Deleuze, G. (1994). *Difference and Repetition* (P. Patton, Trans.). New York: Columbia University Press.

Deleuze, G. (1995). *Negotiations, 1972–1990* (M. Joughin, Trans.). New York: Columbia University Press.

Deleuze, G. (1997). *Essays Critical and Clinical* (D. W. Smith and M. Greco, Trans.). Minneapolis: University of Minnesota Press.

Deleuze, G. (2000). *Proust and Signs* (R. Howard, Trans.). Minneapolis, MN: University of Minnesota Press.

Deleuze, G. (2001). *Pure Immanence: Essays on a Life* (A. Boyman, Trans.). New York: Zone Books.

Deleuze, G. (2003a). *Desert Islands and Other Texts (1953–1974)*. New York: Semiotext(e).

Deleuze, G. (2003b). *Francis Bacon: The Logic of Sensation* (D. W. Smith, Trans.). Minneapolis, MN: University of Minnesota Press.

Deleuze, G. (2007). Mathesis, science and philosophy. In R. Mackay (Ed.), *Collapse III* (pp. 141–55). Falmouth: Urbanomic.

Deleuze, G., and Guattari, F. (1983). *Anti-Oedipus: Capitalism and Schizophrenia* (R. Hurley, M. Seem, and H. R. Lane, Trans.). Minneapolis, MN: University of Minnesota Press.

Deleuze, G., and Guattari, F. (1987). *A Thousand Plateaus: Capitalism and Schizophrenia* (B. Massumi, Trans.). Minneapolis, MN: University of Minnesota Press.

Deleuze, G., and Guattari, F. (1994). *What is Philosophy?* (H. Tomlinson and G. Burchell, Trans.). New York: Columbia University Press.

Deleuze, G., and Parnet, C. (1987). *Dialogues* (H. Tomlinson and B. Habberjam, Trans.). New York: Columbia University Press.

Hederman, M. P. (2003). *Tarot: Talisman or Taboo? Reading the World as Symbol*. Dublin: Currach Press.

Jung, C. G. (1953–1979). *Collected Works* (R. F. C. Hull, Trans.). Princeton, NJ: Princeton University Press. [cited as CW]

Jung, C. G. (1963). *Memories, Dreams, Reflections* (R. Winston and C. Winston, Trans.). New York: Pantheon Books.

Meier, C. A. (Ed.). (2001). *Atom and Archetype: The Pauli/Jung Letters, 1932–1958*. Princeton, NJ: Princeton University Press.

Neumann, E. (1969). *Depth Psychology and a New Ethic* (E. Rolfe, Trans.). London: Hodder and Stoughton.

Pauli, W. (1994). *Writings on Physics and Philosophy* (R. Schlapp, Trans.). Berlin: Springer-Verlag.

Samuels, A. (1985). *Jung and the Post-Jungians*. London and New York: Routledge.

Semetsky, I. (2011). *Re-Symbolization of the Self: Human Development and Tarot Hermeneutic*. Rotterdam: Sense Publishers.

Semetsky, I. (2013). *The Edusemiotics of Images: Essays on the art~science of Tarot*. Rotterdam: Sense Publishers.

Chapter 5

The geometry of wholeness

George Hogenson

A client in my practice, whose artistic skills are highly developed, regularly carries a sketchbook with him in which he draws images from his dreams, paintings and other renderings of his process in analysis. Shortly prior to the conference represented in this book he brought two sketches to our session. The first (Figure 5.1), he recounted, arose spontaneously. When he completed the sketch, he 'sat with it for a long period of time, feeling contented and at peace'.

Several days later he attempted to reproduce the experience, but the figure he drew in this instance left him feeling 'disturbed and unsettled' when he finished (Figure 5.2).

Both images are complex and reward detailed examination, but for purposes of the present discussion I want to focus on the central geometric distinction between them. In the first image we see a centred square that is subdivided into four triangular elements. The quadratic shape itself balances between a space of light — illuminated by a sun-like eye — and complete darkness, while the internal quadratic subdivision demarcates the boundary between the light and dark domains as well as marking their essential conjunction in the vertical. In the second image the central square has been divided into two squares, each of which is subdivided into two triangular elements. The two squares are now balanced within a complex and quite formal structure of incomplete circular patterns, almost mechanical in structure, with the dark element narrowly confined between two of the incomplete circles. The illuminating eye is still present, but like the dark element it appears withdrawn from the central elements of the image, casting only a representation of light, in contrast to the encompassing sense of

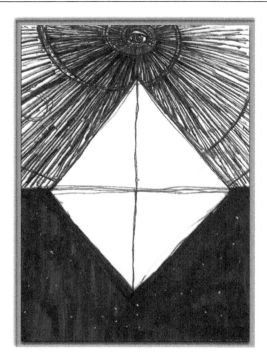

Figure 5.1 Client's first sketch
Reproduced with permission

illumination in the first image. Overall, the image has a highly planned or intentional quality, the result of the artist's desire to recreate an experience that was originally spontaneous.

Jung is clear, and ample phenomenological evidence underwrites his claim, that the most common pattern associated with the experience of wholeness is the quadratic pattern, frequently but not always within a circular structure. These are the classic geometric characteristics of the mandala. Their universality is well attested, ranging from the patterns of Buddhist mandalas such as the Tibetan Kalachakra (Figure 5.3) to the pre-Columbian Aztec such as the Codex Fejérváry-Mayer cosmogram with the fire god Xiuhtecuhtli in the centre (Figure 5.4).

In his essay on mandala symbolism Jung includes a series of mandala figures, some of his own composition and many from his patients, in addition to images from cultural traditions such as the pre-Columbian cosmogram and the Kalachakra. In all of these traditions

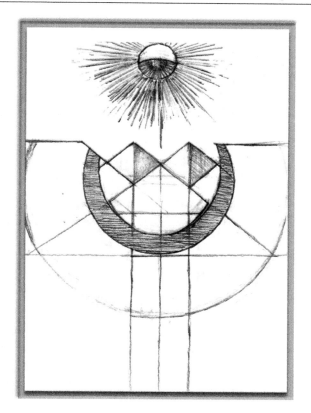

Figure 5.2 Client's second sketch
Reproduced with permission

it is important to keep in mind the correlation that inheres between the cosmographic image and the interior states of those who engage with the mandala. To further set the stage for the argument of this chapter I want to add two more of these mandala-like figures, one from Jung's investigations of the Chinese *I Ching* or *Book of Changes* and the other by a patient following a dream (Figures 5.5 and 5.6).

What is important in these two mandala images is the pattern of quadratic movement either out from a central point or in toward a central point, and the ambiguity as to which direction the pattern is moving. Although Jung's rendering of his patient's mandala is in black and white he reports that it was in fact coloured in red, green, yellow and blue. He goes on to comment that:

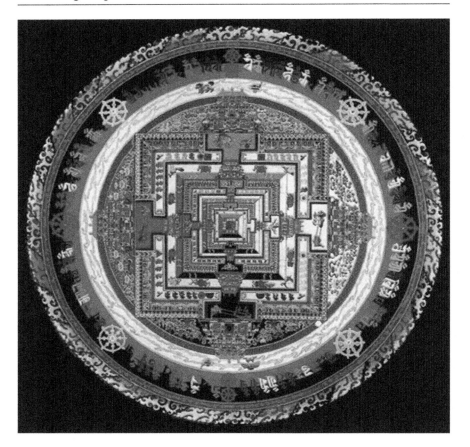

Figure 5.3 Kalachakra mandala
Source: WikiCommons

As to the interpretation of the picture, it must be emphasized that the snake, arranged in angles and then in circles round the square, signifies the circumambulation of, and way to, the centre. The snake, as a chthonic and at the same time spiritual being, symbolizes the unconscious. The stone in the centre, presumably a cube, is the quaternary form of the *lapis philosophorum*. The four colours also point in this direction. It is evident that the stone in this case signifies the new centre of personality, the self, which is also symbolized by a vessel.

(Jung 1969b: §651)

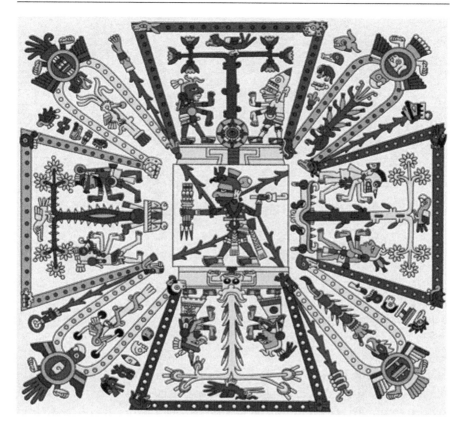

Figure 5.4 Codex Fejérváry-Mayer
Source: WikiCommons

The geometry of wholeness

The question raised by these and many other examples is whether the geometry of the symbolic patterns has a relationship to the experiences associated with them or if they are simply conventional patterns with no deeper significance. Put another way, if we take the two images produced by my client, is there some underlying relationship between the patterns and his experience of peacefulness in the first instance and disturbance in the second? Furthermore, if such a distinction exists, does it tell us something about the experience of wholeness as a psychological phenomenon?

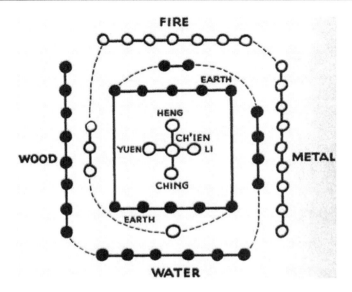

Figure 5.5 'The River Map', one of the legendary foundations of the *I Ching*
Reproduced (with permission) from C. G. Jung, 'Concerning mandala symbolism', Figure 2,
in *Collected Works*, Volume 9i

To work out a possible answer to these questions we can look at what is now recognized as the basic geometry of the natural world, fractal geometry (Mandelbrot 1983). The origins of fractal geometry can be traced back at least to the seventeenth century when mathematicians began to work with recursive patterns. Recursion — the iterative repetition of a simple mathematical process in which the result of one iteration becomes the variable for the next iteration — is central to the generation of fractal patterns. For example, one can draw a straight line down the west coast of Norway, and derive one length for the coastline. It would be immediately evident, however, that this was an unusually inaccurate map. Through a process of recursive fractioning of the original line, however, the map will become increasingly accurate. In principle this process could go on almost infinitely, finally arriving at a map that encompassed even the grains of sand on the shores of the Hardanger Fjord. More illustrative of the formation of fractal patterns are the correspondences that exist between the branching patterns of trees and the vein patterns in the leaves of the tree. Once again, one can see a process of ever-finer reiteration

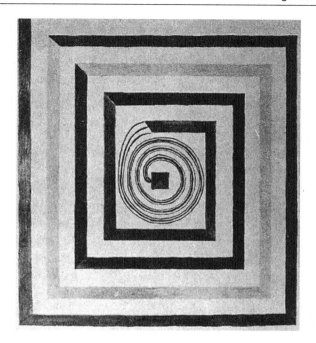

Figure 5.6 Mandala based on a woman's dream
Reproduced (with permission) from C. G. Jung, 'Concerning mandala symbolism', Figure 4, in *Collected Works*, Volume 9i

of a simple recursive structure in the formation of the natural world. Although controversial at extremely large scales, some cosmologists have suggested that the structure of the elusive dark matter follows a fractal pattern, and even that the hypothesized multiverse is fractal in structure.

This last level, while disputed, is at least instructive for purposes of examining the structure of the Kalachakra and Codex Fejérváry-Mayer mandalas, as both of them represent a cosmological map in the form of the domains of the deities who define their structure. The degree to which fractal geometry can subsume phenomena ranging from the structure of neuronal dendrites in the brain to, possibly, the structure of the multiverse was not central to the study of this form of geometry until Benoit Mandelbrot (1924–2010) realized the importance of scaling or the degree to which a phenomenon at one level of scale reproduced itself at ever greater scales. This is the principle that accounts for the self-similarity — another concept in scaling phenomena — between the structure of the tree and the structure of the veins in the tree's leaf. Mandelbrot attributes his discovery of scaling to an accidental reading of a review of a book by the American polymath George Kingsly Zipf (1900–1950), upon the recommendation of his uncle, a distinguished French mathematician.

Zipf was on the faculty of Harvard University, nominally with an appointment in linguistics but with freedom to pursue a variety of interests. He eventually referred to himself as a student of human ecology, by which he meant the entire range of human activity. The research he is best known for, however, involved the scaling phenomena of human institutions, beginning with the size of towns and cities but finally grounding on the frequency of words in texts. What Zipf found was that the relative scale of communities or the frequency of words in a text all followed the same pattern of distribution. If, in a given geographic area, the largest community had 5,000 inhabitants, the next largest community would have approximately 2,500, but there would be two such communities, and so on down to the smallest community. The same relations appear in texts and a variety of other phenomena ranging from the intensity of earthquakes to the frequency of visits to websites on the Internet. Zipf's law, as this phenomenon is now known, is a power law distribution, due to the role of an exponent in the calculation of the pattern, and along with Fibonacci numbers and fractal geometry it seems to be among a small group of calculations that apply to situations that otherwise appear to have no relation to one another.

In a series of papers I have suggested that Zipf's law sheds light on elements of Jung's understanding of symbols and the nature of archetypal phenomena (Hogenson 2004, 2005, 2009, 2014, 2018). The argument in these papers has focused on what I have called symbolic density in which some symbolic structures manifest a deep hermeneutical structure or potential for interpretation. Archetypal phenomena, in this interpretation, are capable of much deeper interpretation than other symbolic structures. This distinction would apply to Jung's critique of Freud's understanding of the symbol as basically a sign, with relatively limited semiotic reference, in distinction to his own understanding of the symbol as referencing otherwise inaccessible dimensions of the psyche.

As with fractals, Zipf's law relies on an iterative process to work out the frequency in the various patterns it describes. I now want to argue that both fractal geometry, as found in Mandelbrot's work and Zipf's theories of scaling, which played a decisive role in the development of Mandelbrot's theorizing, shed light on the geometry of the images associated with wholeness — the mandalas of Jung's patients, Buddhist meditation, and my own client.

The Mandelbrot set

The Mandelbrot set (Figure 5.7) is probably the best-known example of fractal geometry, superseding the Julia set from which it derives much of its structure. The Mandelbrot set was not, however, developed by Mandelbrot but by the French mathematician Adrien Douady, who named the set in honour of Mandelbrot. Much of its fame derives from renderings of the pattern that add colour to certain outcomes of the iterative calculation, $z=z^2+c$. As it happens, the colours that are so captivating are actually outcomes of the equation that fall outside the stipulated boundaries of the set. As one will see in computer-generated renderings of the Mandelbrot set, the patterns that fall outside the original boundaries frequently begin, at a later point in the iterative process, to recapitulate at ever smaller scales, the original pattern of the set. This process of seemingly infinite recursion is one of the most fascinating aspects of the calculation.

It is also the case, however, that the results of the recursive iteration of the formula for the set can be graphed in a variety of forms. The two, to which we will turn our attention here, are known as a bifurcation, or logistic, graph and a cobweb plot or graph. The bifurcation graph typically appears in the form shown in Figure 5.8.

The bifurcations in the graph correspond to critical inflection points on the Mandelbrot set. Essentially, what is happening is that as the formula for the Mandelbrot set evolves, the value of z – in this simplified example – reaches critical points where the graph changes dramatically. If these values are transposed to the bifurcation graph and used as parameter values in that graph, they correspond to critical bifurcation points in the graph, as can be seen in the illustration in Figure 5.9.

The cobweb plot, on the other hand, has the form shown in Figure 5.10.

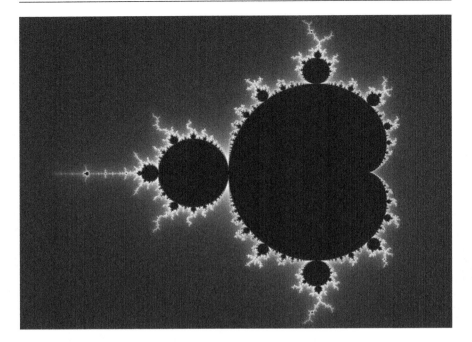

Figure 5.7 The Mandelbrot set
Source: WikiCommons

What interests us here is the relationship between the Mandelbrot set — or, for that matter, other fractal patterns that will fall close to the same graphical outcomes — the bifurcation diagram and the cobweb plot (Figures 5.8, 5.9, and 5.10). Using the same parameters for the calculation in each instance, the graphical depiction of the calculation falls out in distinct patterns, to which we will attend.

In essence, the initial stages of the iterative calculation for the Mandelbrot set results in outcomes that are identical or diverge in only the slightest degree. However, the process of iteration eventually begins to display the characteristics associated with critical dependency on the initial conditions, and divergence occurs abruptly at an inflection point in the graphing process. The initial divergence is a single bifurcation of the plot on the bifurcation graph. This is followed, however, by a further bifurcation, and the eventual emergence of a chaotic regime as the divergences multiply. The point that is of greatest concern to modelling the mandala patterns illustrated above is the first

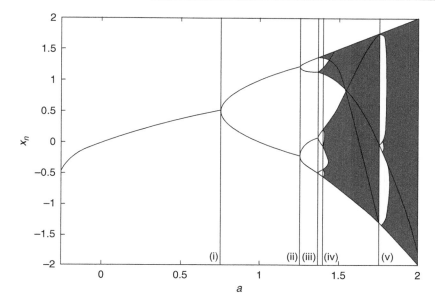

Figure 5.8 Bifurcation graph
Source: WikiCommons

bifurcation. To illustrate this point we can look at a combination of moments in all three graphs (Figures 5.11, 5.12, and 5.13).

Subsequent bifurcations eventually lead to the chaotic regime.[1]

Discussion

Among the themes that are central to Jung's system of psychology, the 'unity of opposites' looms large. Drawing principally from the fifteenth-century Cardinal-philosopher Nicholas of Cusa, Jung's focus is on a variety of unities, such as consciousness and the unconscious or anima and animus. It is in these unities that Jung sees the possibility of an experience of wholeness that he associates with the quadratic form of the mandala:

> Although 'wholeness' seems at first sight to be nothing but an abstract idea (like anima and animus), it is nevertheless empirical in so far as it is anticipated by the psyche in the form of spontane-ous or autonomous symbols. These are the quaternity or mandala

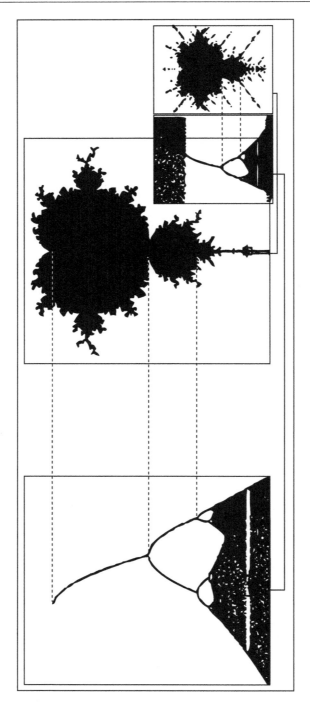

Figure 5.9 Bifurcation and Mandelbrot set
Source: WikiCommons

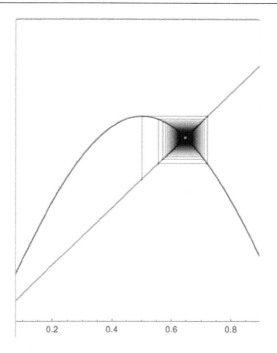

Figure 5.10 Cobweb plot

Source: 'Fractal Geometry', Yale University, Michael Frame, Benoit Mandelbrot (1924–2010), and Nial Neger. Open source.

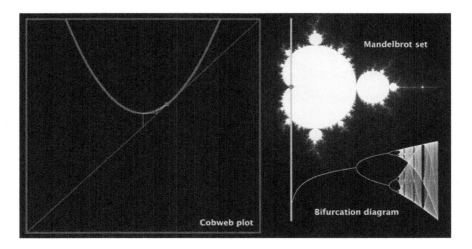

Figure 5.11 The initial stage

Source: Courtesy of Michael Hogg

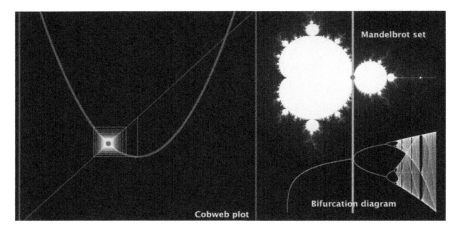

Figure 5.12 The final point of unity
Source: Courtesy of Michael Hogg

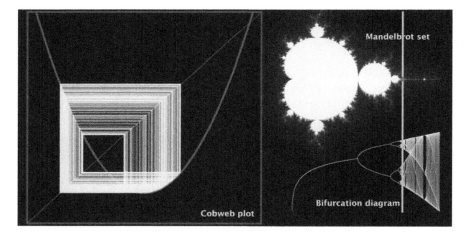

Figure 5.13 Chaos
Source: Courtesy of Michael Hogg

symbols, which occur not only in the dreams of modern people who have never heard of them, but are widely disseminated in the historical records of many peoples and many epochs. Their significance as *symbols of unity and totality* is amply confirmed by history as well as by empirical psychology.

(Jung 1969a: §59)

The other aspect of this view of wholeness, which he derives in part from his study of Gnosticism, is that the quadratic form not only gives shape to psychic wholeness but is imbedded in the material world as well:

> The primordial image of the quaternity coalesces, for the Gnostics, with the figure of the demiurge or Anthropos. He is, as it were, the victim of his own creative act, for, when he descended into Physis, he was caught in her embrace. The image of the anima mundi or Original Man latent in the dark of matter expresses the presence of a transconscious centre which, because of its quaternary character and its roundness, must be regarded as a symbol of wholeness. We may assume, with due caution, that some kind of psychic wholeness is meant (for instance, conscious + unconscious), though the history of the symbol shows that it was always used as a God-image.
>
> (Jung 1969a: §308)

We can now begin to see the possible importance of the relationship between fractal geometry, in our example presented by the Mandelbrot set, and the images of wholeness identified by Jung. The original work done on fractal geometry was confined to the purely mathematical world of Georg Cantor and others, but with Mandelbrot's work and the implementation of fractal geometry on computers it became evident that fractals, in large measure, defined the geometry of the actually existing physical world. If, at the same time, fractals define important elements of the symbolic world of psychic wholeness as conceptualized by Jung it becomes possible to hypothesize a level of psychophysical unity as proposed by Jung, particularly in his collaboration with Wolfgang Pauli.

What we find in the various diagrams presented above is the formation of a quaternity at precisely that point where the first bifurcation occurs, as unity separates into duality. Further progress leads inexorably to a chaotic regime of dispersal, both in the physical world and in the psyche.

Returning then to my client and the two drawings he brought to our session, we can now see that the spontaneously drawn figure that brought with it a sense of calm appears, as a simple quaternity, to occupy that point in the formation of the cobweb plot where unity is on the cusp of bifurcation. The second drawing, intended to recreate the spontaneous experience but failing to do so, occupies the space defined by the bifurcation of unity into duality. A sense of wholeness infuses the first drawing, while the dissonance of duality is reflected in the second. In the same manner we can now see in the cosmic mandalas such as the Kalachakra or the Aztec Codex Fejérváry-Mayer a recognition of the encompassing nature of this inflection point in the geometry of nature and the psyche. Jung saw this correspondence as central to his thinking about synchronicity, remarking on the importance of mathematics as a transcendent aspect of reality:

> Psyche and matter exist in one and the same world, and each partakes of the other, otherwise any reciprocal action would be impossible. If research could only advance far enough, therefore, we should arrive at an ultimate agreement between physical and psychological concepts. Our present attempts may be bold, but I believe they are on the right lines. Mathematics, for instance, has more than once proved that its purely logical constructions which transcend all experience subsequently coincided with the behaviour of things. This, like the events I call synchronistic, points to a profound harmony between all forms of existence.
>
> (Jung 1969a: §413)

The particular mathematics of Jung's own reflections on wholeness, of course, are forms of geometry, and we can now begin to see why the symbolism of wholeness is in fact the form that unifies psyche and physis.

Note

1 The process by which this pattern unfolds can be viewed in its entirety at https://vimeo.com/13566850

References

Hogenson, G. B. (2004). What are symbols symbols of? Situated action, mythological bootstrapping and the emergence of the self. *Journal of Analytical Psychology, 49*(1): 67–81. doi:10.1111/j.0021-8774.2004.0441.x

Hogenson, G. B. (2005). The self, the symbolic and synchronicity: virtual realities and the emergence of the psyche. *Journal of Analytical Psychology*, *50*(3): 271–284. doi:10.1111/j.0021-8774.2005.00531.x

Hogenson, G. B. (2009). Archetypes as action patterns. *Journal of Analytical Psychology*, *54*(3): 325–37. doi:10.1111/j.1468-5922.2009.01783.x

Hogenson, G. B. (2014). Are synchronicities really dragon kings? In H. Atmanspacher & C. A. Fuchs (Eds.), *The Pauli-Jung Conjecture and its Impact Today* (pp. 201–216). Exeter: Imprint Academic.

Hogenson, G. B. (2018). *The Tibetan Book of the Dead* needs work: a proposal for research into the geometry of individuation. In J. Cambray & L. Sawin (Eds.), *Research in Analytical Psychology: Applications from Scientific, Historical, and Cross-Cultural Research* (pp. 172–193). London & New York: Routledge.

Jung, C. G. (1969a). *The Collected Works of C. G. Jung* (Sir H. Read, M. Fordham, & G. Adler, Eds.; W. McGuire, Exec. Ed.; R. F. C. Hull, Trans.) [hereafter *Collected Works*], vol. 9ii, *Aion: Researches Into the Phenomenology of the Self*. London: Routledge & Kegan Paul.

Jung, C. G. (1969b). Concerning mandala symbolism. In *Collected Works,* Vol. 9i, *The Archetypes and the Collective Unconscious*, 355–384. Princeton: Princeton University Press.

Mandelbrot, B. B. (1983). *The Fractal Geometry of Nature*. New York: W. H. Freeman.

Chapter 6

The status of exceptional experiences in the Pauli-Jung conjecture

Harald Atmanspacher

Introduction

Most of our present understanding of mind and its place in nature began to develop around the turn of the twentieth century and, eventually, led to the almost hegemonic pretence of what is today called physicalism. In a nutshell, physicalism claims that nature, including the mind, is essentially described and explained by physics. Typically, physicalist attempts to clarify the nature of mind mean reducing mental states and their behaviour to brain states and their behaviour. Most contemporary neuroscientists adhere, knowingly or not, to this philosophical programme.

There is a variety of versions of physicalism (eliminative, epiphenomenal, reductive, non-reductive, etc.) which I cannot discuss in detail here (see Papineau [2015] for a very brief overview). One crucial assumption in all of them is the so-called 'causal closure (or completeness) of the physical', stating that every event in nature that has a cause has a physical cause. This assumption is widely held without discomfort, though a number of authors have recently expressed concerns about its unquestioned validity (Lowe 2000; Montero 2003; Bishop and Atmanspacher 2011).

However, many of the hopes and promises that the promulgators of the 'decade of the brain' at the turn of the twenty-first century generated are still unfulfilled today. There is no doubt that brain research has yielded important insights, yet an understanding of the fundamental problem of the relationship between our mental lives and what our brains do has surely remained an open problem. The naive idea of one-to-one neural correlates of conscious states has proven pure fantasy (cf. Anderson 2010), and other physicalist-oriented ideas replacing it may turn out difficult to realise as well.

At present we observe that the lack of success of physicalist approaches concerning the solution of one of the deepest questions in the history of mankind, the nature of mind-matter correlations, entails the search for alternative approaches. A most prominent one among those alternatives differs substantially from physicalism and has received increasing attention under the notion of *dual-aspect thinking*.

The historical protagonist of dual-aspect thinking in philosophy is Spinoza, whose conceptual framework addresses the mental and the physical as the two 'attributes' of thought and extension of a psycho-physically neutral substance. For Spinoza, this substance is divine, hence infinite, so that it actually has infinitely many attributes. Only two of them are apperceptible by human beings with their limited intellectual abilities. For this reason, Spinoza's philosophical system belongs to the variety of dual-aspect monisms.[1]

Spinoza's terms of thought and extension suggest that his thinking is a reaction to Descartes' interactive dualism with *res cogitans* and *res extensa*. While this dualism clearly violates the assumption of the causal closure of the physical insofar as it posits that the mental be capable of acting upon the physical, causal closure in Spinoza is violated in a subtler way. Since the attributes, which do not interact directly, derive from one base substance, this substance may inject effects, intrusions as it were, into the attributes. So they are causally closed against one another but not against the psychophysically neutral.

Decompositional dual-aspect monism

Within the tradition of dual-aspect thinking, one can distinguish two different, in a sense opposing, base conceptions.[2] In one of them, psychophysically neutral elementary entities are *composed* into sets of such entities, and depending on the composition these sets acquire mental or physical properties. Major historic proponents of this compositional scheme are Mach, James, Avenarius, and Russell. In the literature, this scheme is often referred to as 'neutral monism' (Stubenberg 2010; Alter and Nagasawa 2012). A much discussed neo-Russellian version of neutral monism has been proposed by Chalmers (1996), which has been quite influential, both in the philosophy of mind and in cognitive neuroscience (cf. the work of Tononi and his group, e.g., Oizumi *et al.* 2014; Tononi 2015; Tononi *et al.* 2016).

The other base conception is closer to Spinoza's original way of thinking, where the psychophysically neutral does not consist of elementary entities waiting to be composed, but is conceived as one overarching whole that is to be *decomposed*. In contrast to the atomistic picture of compositional dual-aspect monism, the holistic picture of the decompositional variant today is strongly reminiscent of the fundamental insight of entanglement in quantum physics. Quantum systems are wholes that can be decomposed in infinitely many complementary ways, very close to how Spinoza's idea of the divine has been interpreted.

Inspired by its quantum theoretical significance, modern decompositional dual-aspect thinking has been mainly proposed by philosophically oriented physicists in the twentieth century, starting with Bohm and Pauli (together with the psychologist C. G. Jung). Subsequent work along the same lines has been due to d'Espagnat, Primas, and others. A key difference between compositional and decompositional accounts is that the mental and the physical are reducible to neutral elements if these are the basis for composition, but they are irreducible (in the standard understanding of reduction) to a neutral whole if this is the basis for decomposition.

A second important point is that decomposition necessarily implies correlations between the emerging parts, while composition does not necessarily give rise to correlations between different sets of composed elements. In this way, decompositional dual-aspect monism has been highlighted as the one philosophical framework that explains mental-physical correlations most elegantly and naturally. The price to be paid is that the metaphysics of a psychophysically neutral whole is largely undeveloped and leaves much work to be done. We will present a speculative approach toward successive layers of decomposition in terms of symmetry breakings and resulting partitions below in the section on 'Consciousness and the unconscious in the mental domain'.

One additional piece of support for the decompositional picture derives from the distinction of ontic and epistemic levels of reality, which has been successfully employed in the interpretation of quantum physics (Atmanspacher and Primas 2003). The leading analogy here is that an ultimately undivided ontic universe of discourse is epistemically inaccessible since it offers no distinctions. Successive decompositions introduce more and more refined layers that can be epistemically (e.g. cognitively, or otherwise empirically) accessed.

The decompositional version of dual-aspect monism suggested by Pauli and Jung (cf. Atmanspacher 2012 for an overview with many original references) offers interesting options to explore such refined layers through Jung's concept of archetypes, somewhat analogous to the basic symmetry breakings that governed the early evolution of the fundamental interactions in the physical universe.

The Pauli-Jung conjecture

Pauli and Jung began to think about mind-matter relations fairly soon after they first met in 1932, but the intense interaction that led to their version of dual-aspect monism happened after Pauli's return from Princeton to Zurich in 1946. Their discussions were accompanied by an extensive exchange of ideas that Pauli had with his colleague Fierz at Basel. Fortunately, much of this material is today accessible (in German) in von Meyenn's masterful eight-volume edition of Pauli's correspondence.

Although neither Pauli nor Jung was much inclined to discuss their ideas with contemporary academic philosophers (aside from a few exceptions), their conversations had a distinctly philosophical flavour. However, their usage of philosophical concepts and notions was

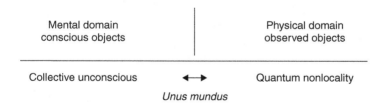

Figure 6.1 According to the Pauli-Jung conjecture, the mental and the physical are manifestations of an underlying, psychophysically neutral, holistic reality, called *unus mundus*, whose symmetry must be broken to yield dual, complementary aspects. From the mental, the neutral reality is approached via Jung's collective unconscious; from the physical, it is approached via quantum nonlocality.

unsystematic. It was typical for them to avail themselves of the history of philosophy as they saw something fit their position or intention. Nevertheless, their comprehensive correspondence yields valuable information, allowing a coherent and detailed reconstruction of their approach: the *Pauli-Jung conjecture* (Atmanspacher and Fuchs 2014).

In the following I will sketch the framework of the Pauli-Jung version of decompositional dual-aspect monism (depicted by the cartoon in Figure 6.1) in four parts: (1) the relation between local realism and holism in quantum physics, (2) the relation between consciousness and the unconscious in Jung's psychology, (3) the common, psychophysically neutral ground of both the mental, conscious realm and the physical, local realm, and (4) the relation between these realms as a consequence of and mediated by their common ground.

Local realism and holism in the physical domain

Today there is wide agreement that the fundamental theory of physical matter is quantum theory. Yet one of its central problems, perhaps the most difficult one, is a proper understanding of the process of measurement. Although much progress has been achieved toward its solution since the early days of quantum mechanics, the measurement problem is still not completely understood. However, empirical results and modern formulations of quantum theory allow us to state it in a way that is more precise than ever before.

A measurement process can be viewed as an intervention decomposing the state of a so-called entangled system, for example the state Φ_{pair} of a *photon pair*. This pair state is *not* the same as the product of the states Φ_1 and Φ_2 of *two separate photons*; we write this as $\Phi_{pair} \neq \Phi_1 \otimes \Phi_2$. The two photon states arise from the pair state as soon as a property of the system, like spin, is measured: $\Phi_{pair} \rightarrow \Phi_1 \otimes \Phi_2$. The decomposition of the entangled state Φ_{pair} into local states Φ_1 and Φ_2 abolishes the former state Φ_{pair} of the system as a whole and entails nonlocal correlations between its disentangled parts, the two photon states. These nonlocal correlations are *not* created by causal signals between the two photons. They are due to the holistic nature of the pair state from which they arise.

Conceptually speaking, measurement is the transition from an unobserved state to observed states of a system. At the same time it suppresses the connectedness constituting a holistic reality and generates separate local objects constituting a local reality. This issue of empirical access is mirrored by the important philosophical difference of ontic and epistemic states. Ontic states and associated intrinsic properties refer to the holistic concept of reality, are operationally inaccessible, and are supposed to characterise the system independent of its observation and our resulting knowledge. In contrast, epistemic states and associated contextual properties refer to a local concept of a reality that is operationally accessible by measurement (and observation).[3]

In the framework of algebraic quantum theory, the ontic-epistemic distinction can be mathematically formalised and has turned out to be powerful and attractive for understanding the differences and similarities of various interpretational schemes in quantum theory. A helpful source for more details in this regard is a comprehensive account of epistemic and ontic quantum realities by Atmanspacher and Primas (2003). Today we know that both state concepts, the ontic and the epistemic, are together necessary for a comprehensive description of reality; neither of them is sufficient on its own.[4]

One may wonder why it is useful to have an ontic level of description at which direct empirical (or operational) access is no option in principle. However, a most appealing feature of an ontic description is that it comprises first principles and universal laws that are unavailable in a purely epistemic description. From a proper ontic description it is possible to deduce proper epistemic descriptions, given enough details – contexts as it were – are known about the epistemic (empirical) framework that is at stake.

Although this is a fairly modern picture, it also has a conservative aspect: quantum theory as of today does not at any place refer to the mental world of human observers, to their cognitive capabilities or psychological condition. Any inanimate environment can play the role of a 'measuring device', though in a non-intentional manner. No consciousness is necessary for measuring a quantum state. On the other hand, as soon as *controlled* experiments are considered, it is clear that issues like the design of an experiment, the choice of observables of interest, or the interpretation of the results of a measurement are crucial. They depend on decisions based on the intentions of human observers and *are not part of the formalism of quantum theory*.

In a letter to Fierz of August 10, 1954 (von Meyenn 1999: 742–747, translation HA), Pauli speculated:

> It might be that matter, for instance considered from the perspective of life, is not treated 'properly' if it is observed as in quantum mechanics, *namely totally neglecting the inner state of the 'observer'*. [...] The well-known 'incompleteness' of quantum mechanics (Einstein) is certainly an existing fact somehow-somewhere, but of course it cannot be removed by reverting to classical field physics (that is only a 'neurotic misunderstanding' of Einstein), it has much more to do with *holistic relationships between 'inside' and 'outside' which contemporary science does not contain*.

In his privately distributed manuscript on 'modern examples of background physics', Pauli (1948) emphasised that the measurement problem 'does not indicate an incompleteness of quantum theory within physics but an incompleteness of physics within the totality of life'. Pauli's uneasiness with the status of science in general and physics in particular was not an odd idea but a serious criticism of great relevance. The question is how to turn it into viable research.

Consciousness and the unconscious in the mental domain

According to the Pauli-Jung conjecture, the role which measurement plays as a link between local and holistic realities in physics is mirrored by the act in which subjects become consciously aware of 'local mental objects', as it were, arising from holistic unconscious contents in psychology. The holistic realities of physics and psychology project in parallel onto mental and physical local realities. This idea is most clearly elaborated in Jung's supplement to his 'On the nature of the psyche' (Jung 1969).[5] Here is a quote from a letter by Pauli that Jung cites in footnote 130 in this supplement (ibid.: §439):

> [...] the epistemological situation regarding the concepts of 'consciousness' and the 'unconscious' seems to offer a close analogy to the situation of 'complementarity' in physics, sketched below. On the one hand, the unconscious can only be made accessible in an indirect way by its (ordering) influence on conscious contents, on

the other hand every 'observation of the unconscious', i.e. every attempt to make unconscious contents conscious, has a *prima facie* uncontrollable reaction back onto these unconscious contents themselves (as is well known, this precludes that the unconscious can be 'exhaustively' brought to consciousness). The physicist will *per analogiam* conclude that precisely this uncontrollable backlash of the observing subject onto the unconscious limits the objective character of its reality and, at the same time, provides it with some subjectivity. [...] The development of 'microphysics' has unmistakably led to a remarkable convergence of its description of nature with that of the new psychology: while the former, due to the fundamental situation known as 'complementarity', faces the impossibility to eliminate actions of observers by determinable corrections and must therefore in principle relinquish the objective registration of all physical phenomena, the latter could basically complement the merely subjective psychology of consciousness by postulating the existence of an unconscious of largely objective reality.

It is important to realise that the relation between holistic and local realms in both mental and physical domains is conceived as *bidirectional*. Unconscious contents can become conscious, and simultaneously this very transition changes the unconscious left behind. Analogously, physical measurement necessitates a decomposition of the holistic realm, and simultaneously this very measurement changes the state of the system left behind. This picture, already outlined in Pauli's letter to Fierz of October 3, 1951 (von Meyenn 1996: 377), represents a genuine interdependence between holistic and local domains. It can entail *indirect* mind–matter correlations via the holistic realm that occur in addition to those correlations that are due to dual epistemic 'manifestations' of that realm.

In the same context, Jung (1969: §439) makes a significant move away from his previous understanding of archetypes as (biological) hereditary instincts over (psychological) raw feelings and inner images to the more advanced notion of psychophysically neutral, transcendental (or metaphysical) principles. Since his mature understanding of archetypes embraces both their manifestations in subjective consciousness and their origin in the impersonal objective unconscious,

Jung invented the term 'psychoid' to characterise them as structural principles beyond the conscious psyche.

Archetypes and unus mundus

The simple but radical idea of the Pauli-Jung conjecture is the assumption of a background reality from which the mental and the physical are supposed to emerge as epistemically distinguishable. Although physics and psychology point to their common basis in different ways, the basis itself is assumed to be of unitary nature: a psychophysically neutral domain that is neither mental nor physical, a *tertium quid*.

Already in 1948, Pauli expressed his predilection for such a psychophysically neutral domain beneath (or beyond) the mental and the physical in a letter to Fierz of 7 January 1948 (von Meyenn 1993: 496f, translation HA):

> *The ordering and regulating factors must be placed beyond the distinction of 'physical' and 'psychic'* – as Plato's 'ideas' share the notion of a concept and of a force of nature (they create actions out of themselves). I am very much in favour of referring to the 'ordering' and 'regulating' factors in terms of 'archetypes'; but then it would be inadmissible to *define* them as contents of the *psyche*. The mentioned inner images ('dominant features of the collective unconscious' after Jung) are rather *psychic* manifestations of the archetypes which, *however*, would *also* have to put forth, create, condition anything law-like in the behaviour of the corporeal world. The laws of this world would then be the *physical manifestations of the archetypes*. [...] *Each* law of nature should then have an inner correspondence and vice versa, even though this is not always directly visible today.

Jung's psychology hosts quite a selection of archetypes, to which different degrees of unconscious depth can be ascribed. Among Jungians there is agreement that the shadow and the anima/animus complex are the first and therefore least deep-seated archetypes with whose manifestations individuals become confronted. Candidates for more fundamental archetypes are the self, as the goal of the individuation process, and maybe most basic the archetype of number, expressing qualitative principles like unity, duality, trinity, quaternity, and so forth.

The term Jung used for the ultimately ontic, psychophysically neutral domain without any distinctions is the *unus mundus*, the one world, a notion adopted from the 16th-century Belgian physician and alchemist Gerardus Dorneus. In his *Mysterium Coniunctionis* of 1955–56, Jung writes (1970: §767):

> Undoubtedly the idea of the *unus mundus* is founded on the assumption that the multiplicity of the empirical world rests on an underlying unity, and that not two or more fundamentally different worlds exist side by side or are mingled with one another. Rather, everything divided and different belongs to one and the same world, which is not the world of sense but a postulate [...].

Divisions or distinctions are a basic principle of every epistemology, sometimes called an epistemic split. In somewhat more abstract terms, distinctions can be conceived as symmetry breakings. Symmetries in this parlance are invariances under transformations.[6] An entirely distinction-free, totally symmetric state of affairs is associated with a radically undivided reality, to which there is no epistemic access at all.

When the holistic *unus mundus* is split, correlations emerge between the resulting domains. These correlations are remnants, as it were, of the wholeness that is lost due to the distinction made. Splitting the *unus mundus* as the holistic domain into mental and physical domains suggests ubiquitous correlations between mental and physical states.

Mind–matter correlations and synchronicity

Conceiving the mind–matter distinction in terms of splitting a psychophysically neutral domain implies correlations between mind and matter as a direct and generic consequence. It is important, though, to stress that these correlations are not due to causal interactions (in the sense of efficient causation as usually looked for in science) between the mental and the physical. In the Pauli-Jung conjecture it would be wrong to interpret mind (or mental states) as caused by matter (or physical states) or vice versa.

Pauli and Jung discussed such correlations extensively in their correspondence between June 1949 and February 1951 when Jung drafted his article on *synchronicity* for the book that he published jointly with Pauli (Jung and Pauli 1955). A mental and a physical event, apparently accidental and not necessarily simultaneous, are called synchronistic if they are neither causally related nor pure chance, but correspond with one another by their joint meaning.

Pauli and Jung thought that synchronistic phenomena cannot be corroborated by statistical methods as they are usually applied in the sciences. In a letter to Fierz of 3 June 1952, Pauli wrote (von Meyenn 1996: 634f, translation HA) that:

> synchronistic phenomena [...] elude being captured in natural 'laws' since they are not reproducible, i.e. unique, and are blurred by the statistics of large numbers. By contrast, 'acausalities' in physics are precisely described by statistical laws (of large numbers).

And in his 'Lecture to the foreign people' (Atmanspacher et al. 1995: 326, translation HA), where Pauli sketched some of his ideas about biological evolution, he stated that:

> *external physical circumstances on the one hand and corresponding adaptive hereditary alterations of genes (mutations) on the other are not connected causally-reproducibly, but occur – correcting the 'blind' chance fluctuations of the mutations – meaningfully and purposefully as inseparable wholes together with the external circumstances.* According to this hypothesis, which differs from both Darwin's and Lamarck's conception, we encounter the requested *third type* of natural laws, *consisting of corrections of the fluctuations of chance due to meaningful or purposeful coincidences of non-causally connected events.*

What Pauli here postulates is a kind of lawful regularity beyond both deterministic and statistical laws, based on the notion of *meaning* and, thus, clearly not a subject of physics proper. In modern philosophy of mind, meaning is covered by the term 'intentionality', and it is understood as a reference relation between a representation and what it represents (cf. Atmanspacher and Fach 2019 for more details).

However, meaning in this sense is also not a subject of psychology proper. It is a relational concept, relating a mental representation to objects in the physical world. Therefore, synchronistic events, constituted by the joint meaning of mental and physical states, are paradigm examples of mind–matter correlations, or psychophysical correlations. They result from the epistemic split, or symmetry breakdown, differentiating the mental and the physical, and they express the undivided wholeness of the *unus mundus* from which they derive.

There is a stunning analogy of this picture to physical entanglement sketched above in the section on 'Local realism and holism in the physical domain': just replace Φ_{pair} with the psychophysically neutral domain and Φ_1 and Φ_2 with the mental and the physical. While physical correlations between two photon states Φ_1 and Φ_2 are purely *statistical* though, correlations between the mental and the physical comprise both objective and subjective elements: they are *meaningful*.

At this point it may be interesting to inject that Deleuze, in his studies of Jung in relation to Spinoza, makes the following observation (Deleuze 1999: 326–27):

> One feels that the soul and body have at once a sort of identity that removes the need for any real causality between them, and a heterogeneity, a heteronomy, that renders it impossible. The identity or quasi-identity is an 'invariance', and the heteronomy is that between two varying series, one of which is corporeal, the other spiritual. Now real causality enters into each of these series on their own account; but the relation between the two series, and their relation to what is invariant between them, depends on non-causal correspondence. If we then ask what concept can account for such a correspondence, that of expression appears to do so [...], since it brings a correspondence and a resonance into series that are altogether foreign to one another.

Deleuze here relates non-causal correspondence to a resonance expressing the identity of the invariant ground of the mental and the physical. It is an expression of the origin of the experience of meaning, not an expression of a cause by its effect, as in what he calls real causality. In the Pauli-Jung conjecture, this is what synchronicities are all about. Moreover, archetypes and their role in manifesting synchronicities suggest a distinction between two basic kinds of psychophysical correlations for which we have proposed the notions of 'structural' and 'induced' correlations (Atmanspacher and Fach 2013).

Structural correlations refer to the role of archetypes as ordering factors with a *unidirectional* influence on the mental and the physical (Pauli's letter to Fierz of 1948, von Meyenn 1993: 496–97). They arise due to the epistemic split of the psychophysically neutral domain, generating mental and physical aspects. Structural correlations are a straightforward consequence of the basic structure of dual-aspect monism. They are assumed to be persistent and empirically reproducible.

Induced correlations refer to the back-reaction that changes of consciousness induce in the unconscious and, via the unidirectional correlations, in the physical world as well. (Likewise, measurements of physical systems induce back-reactions in the physical ontic reality, which can lead to changes of mental states.) This way, the picture is extended to a *bidirectional* framework of thinking (Pauli's letter to Jung of 1954, Jung 1969: §439). In contrast to structural, persistent correlations, induced correlations depend on all kinds of contexts. They occur only occasionally and are evasive and not (easily) reproducible.

While structural correlations define a baseline of ordinary, robust psychophysical correlations (such as mind–brain correlations or psychosomatic correlations), induced correlations (positive or negative) may be responsible for deviations above or below this baseline. Induced positive correlations, above the baseline, are characterised as phenomena with *excess correlations* – similar to 'salience' phenomena (cf. Kapur 2003). Synchronistic events clearly belong to this class. Induced negative correlations, below the baseline, are characterised as phenomena with *deficit correlations*.

Again, in both induced and structural correlations there is no direct causal relation from the mental to the physical or vice versa (i.e. no direct 'efficient causation'). The problem of a direct 'causal interaction' between the categorically distinct regimes of the mental and the physical is thus avoided. Of course, this does not mean that the correlations themselves have no reason: the origin of structural correlations is the epistemic split of the psychophysically neutral domain. The origin of induced correlations is interventions in the conscious mental or in the physical domain, whose back-effects on the psychophysically neutral level manifest themselves in the complementary domain, respectively.

Exceptional experiences

Phenomenological typology

Experiences are called ordinary if they are consistent with typical *models of reality* that individuals develop to cope with their environment. In modern societies, basic elements of such models are established epistemological concepts (such as cause-and-effect relations) and scientific principles and laws (such as gravitation). Experiences inconsistent with those basic elements or deviating from them are considered exceptional (see Fach *et al.* 2013 for more details).

Two fundamental components within the global model of reality of individuals are the *self-model* and the *world-model*. The distinction between them may seem to resemble the Cartesian distinction of *res cogitans* and *res extensa*, but there is a decisive difference: while Descartes' dualism is ontologically conceived, both self-model and world-model in the Pauli-Jung conjecture are explicitly epistemic.

The world-model contains representations of states of the material world, including the individual's own bodily features. The referents of these representations are observationally accessible and provide intersubjective knowledge, sometimes called 'objective' or 'third-person' knowledge. The self-model contains representations of internal mental states, such as sensations, cognitions, volitions, affects, motivations, inner images. As a rule, these states can only be experienced by the individual itself – they are 'subjective' and based on 'first-person' accounts.

World-model and self-model are often experienced as correlated. For instance, the bodily organs or limbs, representations in an individual's world-model, and bodily sensations, representations in an individual's self-model, are usually experienced in strong mutual relationship. Nevertheless, an individual can distinguish self and world. Mental states induced by external sensory stimuli differ from states generated by internal processing. Individuals are usually capable of differentiating their inner images, affects and fantasies from their perception of physical events in their world-model.

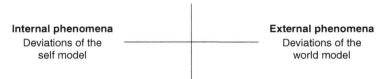

Coincidence phenomena
Connection of ordinarily disconnected elements
of self model and world model

Internal phenomena
Deviations of the
self model

External phenomena
Deviations of the
world model

Dissociation phenomena
Disconnection of ordinarily connected elements
of self model and world model

Figure 6.2 Four fundamental classes of exceptional experiences resulting from the conceptual framework of the Pauli-Jung conjecture

Exceptional experiences (EEs) typically appear as deviations[7] in an individual's reality model. This entails a classification of EEs based on two pairs of phenomena (cf. Fach 2011). One pair refers to deviating experiences within the subject's self-model and world-model, while the other refers to the way in which elements of those models are merged or separated above or below ordinary ('baseline') correlations. This results in four classes of EE (see also Figure 6.2).

1. *External phenomena* are experienced in the world-model. They include visual, auditory, tactile, olfactory, and kinetic phenomena, the impression of invisible but present agents, inexplicable bodily changes, phenomena concerning audio or visual recordings or the location or structure of physical objects.
2. *Internal phenomena* are experienced in the self-model. They include somatic sensations, unusual moods and feelings, thought insertion, inner voices, and intriguing inner images. As in class (1), the affected individual is convinced that familiar explanations are suspended, and the experiences appear ego-dystonic.
3. *Coincidence phenomena* refer to experiences of relations between self-model and world-model that are not founded on regular senses or bodily functions, but instead exhibit connections between ordinarily disconnected elements of the self-model and world-model. Typically, these *excess correlations* are assumed to be non-causal,

often experienced as a salient or meaningful link between mental and physical events.[8]

4. *Dissociation phenomena* are manifested by disconnections of ordinarily connected elements of self-model and world-model. For instance, individuals are not in full control of their bodies, or experience autonomous behaviour not deliberately set into action. Sleep paralysis, out-of-body experiences,[9] and various forms of automatised behaviour are among the most frequent phenomena in this class, which is characterised by *deficit correlations*.

Atmanspacher and Fach (2013, 2019), Fach *et al.* (2013) and Fach (2020) showed how this classification is backed up by comprehensive empirical material. This is not the place to go into details about this. Let me just state that an overall number of over 2300 cases of EEs documented at the Institute for Frontier Areas of Psychology and Mental Health (IGPP) at Freiburg and currently six surveys based on questionnaires for different groups of again more than 2300 individuals confirmed the proposed classification impressively.

Transcendence or immanence?

As mentioned above, EEs of the two pairs of phenomena have different status. While EEs in classes (1) and (2) refer to internal and external phenomena, i.e. to deviations of the self-model and the world-model themselves, classes (3) and (4) refer to *relations* between them. EEs in (1) and (2) are typically reported as categorially *reified* with respect to self or world. EEs in (3) and (4) are basically *relational* between self and world, although their experience is often described in reified terms belonging to self or world or both.

A synchronistic experience, for instance, is not experienced as such unless the *link* between a mental state and the physical state to which it corresponds is experienced. It was Jung's brilliant move to postulate the experience of *meaning* as this link. In a way, this experience of meaning can be regarded as our 'sense' of psychophysical correlations, as the ordinary senses refer to ordinary perception. By postulating meaning as a relational experience, Jung makes explicit that he addresses something beyond physics and psychology. And by excluding causality and chance he goes beyond the two reflexes that the explanatory reper-toire of physicalism offers for observed correlations.

Both Pauli and Jung insisted that archetypes and anything else below the horizontal line in Figure 6.1 are not empirically accessible in any direct way. Yet, since the psychophysically neutral domain below the line mediates between and impacts on the mental and the physical, it can generate manifestations that deliver indirect information about itself. This way of thinking is very much in the Kantian spirit of a *transcendental* realm containing the conditions for the possibility of experiences occurring in empirical reality. The transcendental itself remains inaccessible.

But this position is not canonical. There is a long tradition of so-called mystical experiences that are neither reified nor relational, but rather *immanent*.[10] The classic work by Stace (1960) extracted some elementary features of mystical experiences from various spiritual tra-ditions, some of which also relate to dreams: unification of opposites; no distinction between mental and physical; no spatial or temporal localisation; intense emotion of peace, joy, bliss, blessedness, lucidity or light; awareness beyond ordinary mental functions. Marshall (2005) provides a more recent, very readable and detailed study of mystical experiences.

Mystical experiences are hard to communicate in conventional lan-guage and logic, and corresponding attempts often result in *paradoxi-cal* formulations (Bagger 2007). Opposite notions such as good and evil can emerge as simultaneous representations of an underlying iden-tity in the sense of a *coincidence of opposites*, a big theme of the Neo-Platonist Nicolas of Cusa (Miller 2013) and adopted by Jung. Also in the terminology of Jung (1953), the many facets of the individual ego (first-person singular, with its first-person perspective) are seen as representations of an overarching archetypal *self* that unfolds itself in the process of *individuation*.

Adopting a notion introduced by Gebser (1986), we proposed char-acterising these types of experiences as 'acategorial' (Atmanspacher 1992; Atmanspacher and Fach 2005), referring to states that are expe-rienced without conceptual, or categorial, content (see Gunther 2003; Feil and Atmanspacher 2010). The difficulties in communicating these experiences, as those of acategorial states in general, often lead to met-aphorical descriptions in which categorial terms are used to indicate what has been experienced acategorially. One way to do this amounts to reifying projections onto physical objects or mental images.

An example: experiences of joy, bliss and lucidity are often referred to as experiences of 'light'. However, it would be a naive misunderstanding to interpret such experiences as an electromagnetic field within the body. And it would be equally misguided to interpret them in terms of a merely mental image of light. The mystic sees them as ultimately transcending the distinction between self and world, inside and outside, subject and object. Marshall (2005: 24) has an impressive example of a light experience that starts relational, that is, between inside and outside, and becomes immanent, that is, transcends that distinction:

> I suddenly found myself surrounded, embraced, by a white light, which seemed both to come from within and from without, a very bright light but quite unlike any ordinary physical light. [...] I had the feeling of being 'one' with everything and 'knowing' all things. [...] I had the sense of this being utter Reality, the real Real, far more real and vivid than the ordinary everyday 'reality' of the physical world.

If one trusts the sources, it is crucial for such experiences to be stupendous experiences of numinosity. We may assume that such experiences actually belong neither to the physical nor to the mental realm, nor are they relations between the two as in experienced meaning. If meaning is a relation explicated through an epistemic mind–matter split, immanent experiences point right to the psychophysically neutral source of explicate meaning. They are non-discursive yet open to experience. But careful: without the epistemic split of subject and object, such experiences cannot be subjective in the usual sense of a first-person experience any more!

Mysterium coniunctionis

At the end of his life, Jung published his last major work, which is also his final account on alchemy: *Mysterium Coniunctionis* (1970). At the end of this book we find several sections in Chapter VI, in which he explains his eventual understanding of the alchemical *coniunctio*, the coincidence of opposites. And here we find his last great move, enlarging his framework of thinking from his previous neo-Kantian stance of an inaccessible transcendence to the direct experience of immanence.

Jung's account of the *coniunctio* is essentially based on his reading of Gerardus Dorneus (also known as Gerhard Dorn) whom we met before, a follower and promulgator of the ideas and scriptures of Paracelsus. One of Dorn's most important works was his *Speculativa Philosophia*, part two of his *Clavis Totius Philosophiae Chymisticae* of 1567.[11] Dorn, and with him Jung, distinguishes three successive stages or degrees of the *coniunctio*.

The first of them, the *unio mentalis*, aims – roughly speaking – at the emergence of the self from the ego in the process of individuation, in other words: toward self-awareness. Jung (1970: §707) writes:

> In the language of hermetic philosophy, the conscious ego-personality's coming to terms with its own background, the so-called shadow, corresponds to the union of spirit and soul in the *unio mentalis*, which is the first stage of the *coniunctio*. The extreme opposition of the shadow to consciousness is mitigated by complementary and compensatory processes in the unconscious.

Elsewhere Jung expresses that the shadow is just the first encounter with elements of the unconscious, of which others have to follow in order to complete the process (see also the section above on 'Archetypes and *unus mundus*').

In the second stage, the integrated mind (*unio mentalis*) is to become united with the bodily sphere, respectively with the corporeal world in general. This refers directly to the mind–matter problem. At the second-stage *coniunctio*, relations between the mental and the physical are explicitly experienced. While there is always a temptation to project these experiences into the mental or the physical, they must be understood as *relational, not reified*.[12] This is where Jung (1970: §662, translation HA) places the relevance of synchronistic phenomena:

> Although synchronistic phenomena occur in time and space, they are remarkably independent of these two indispensable determinants of physical existence and do not conform to the law of

causality in our scientific worldview. Its tendency to carefully separate all parallel events from one another is absolutely necessary for reliable scientific knowledge, but it also loosens and obscures the universal connectedness of events. This in turn renders any insight into the *unity of the world* more and more difficult.

Only if the second-stage *coniunctio* is accomplished does the possibility of the most comprehensive third-stage *coniunctio* arise: the unification with and in the *unus mundus* (Jung 1970: §760 translation HA):

> The one and simple is what Dorneus called the *unus mundus*. This one world was the *res simplex*. For him, the third and highest degree of the *coniunctio* was the union of the integrated human with the *unus mundus* – the potential world of the first day of creation, when nothing was yet *in actu*, no two or many, but just one.

Jung uses his terms carefully: *res simplex*, the eternal ground of all empirical being as the merger of *res cogitans* and *res extensa*; potentiality in contrast to actuality, so that we may speak of the reality of both the possible and the actual; and the first day of creation as the undivided oneness from which the multifaceted diversity of the empirical world emerges.

The *mysterium coniunctionis* is the alchemist's formula, and Jung's eventual testimony, for experiences that transcend the distinction of the mental and the physical and point toward their common ground. Yet the mysterium can be experienced as *immanent*, as such, not only as a metaphysical speculation of our cognitive minds.

Acknowledgements

This article contains material adapted from previous publications in the *Journal of Consciousness Studies 19*(9) (2012): 96–120, and in *Mind and Matter 15* (2017): 111–129, with permission by author and editors.

Notes

1 Spinoza was well received by the German idealists (Hegel: 'philosophy is Spinozist or it's no philosophy at all'), and a number of other important

figures in the history of philosophy, such as Schopenhauer, Avenarius, James, Whitehead, and Russell remind us of Spinoza's dual-aspect thinking. Its more recent renaissance in philosophy is exemplified by philosophers such as Brüntrup, Chalmers, Deleuze, Nagel, Sayre, Seager, Strawson, and others. Philosophically interested physicists with a dual-aspect account are Mach, Pauli, Bohm and, more recently, Polkinghorne, Lockwood, d'Espagnat, Primas, and Haken. Of particular interest are variants of dual-aspect thinking in psychology. Pertinent names are Fechner, Jung (together with Pauli), and currently Velmans, Damasio, Solms, Panksepp, Hobson, Friston, and the much discussed approach by Tononi.

2 A compact account of twentieth-century examples of these conceptions can be found in Atmanspacher (2014), including commentaries by Horst, Seager, and Silberstein.

3 It should be noted that David Bohm's version of aspect monism offers a one-to-one parallel to the ontic–epistemic distinction with his distinction of implicate and explicate orders (see Atmanspacher 2014 for discussion). Murphy (1998) discusses how Bohm's terminology translates into the conceptual framework that the French philosopher Deleuze (1994) proposed. His distinction is between the virtual and the actual, which together constitute reality. With these terms Deleuze counters the opposition of possibility (or potentiality) versus reality that has been prominent in some interpretations of quantum theory. On Deleuze's view, the possible is already part of reality, not a precursor to reality from which it unfolds.

4 In a more comprehensive picture, the concepts of epistemic and ontic states need to be considered relative to a chosen descriptive framework. This leads to the notion of relative onticity introduced by Atmanspacher and Kronz (1999).

5 The German original was first published as 'Der Geist der Psychologie' in 1946, and later revised and expanded (including the supplement) as 'Theoretische Überlegungen zum Wesen des Psychischen' in 1954.

6 For instance, the curvature of a circle is invariant under rotations by any arbitrary angle. A circle thus exhibits complete rotational symmetry. Symmetry breakings are a powerful mathematical tool in large parts of theoretical physics, but we do not know better than by pure speculation which symmetries are to be ascribed to the *unus mundus*.

7 Such deviations are often referred to as 'anomalies', or 'paranormal', 'psychic' or 'psi' experiences. We prefer the notion of a deviation because the theoretical approach taken here entails basic classes of such deviations that can be systematically distinguished. This renders the term 'anomalies' (in the sense of singular unsystematic occurrences) to be at least arguable – if not inappropriate.

8 Meaningful coincidences such as 'synchronicities' à la Jung (1972) are examples, including extrasensory perception and related phenomena.

9 Metzinger (2005) provides a challenging discussion of out-of-body experiences based on the concept of phenomenal models of intentionality relations. See also Atmanspacher and Fach (2019).

10 It is not accidental that Deleuze coined the notion of immanence as the 'vertigo of philosophy', vividly discussed and meticulously analysed by Kerslake (2002). See also his more general account in Kerslake (2007).

11 Dorn's *Speculative Philosophy* has been translated by Paul Ferguson and is available through Adam McLean's alchemy website at www.alchemyweb-site.com/bookshop/mohs34.html.

12 Jung discusses the reification of the relational at length, for instance when he criticises the misplaced concreteness sometimes ascribed to alchemical symbols, such as the lapis as a physical body that can be produced in the laboratory.

References

Alter, T. and Nagasawa, Y. (2012). What is Russellian monism? *Journal of Consciousness Studies 19*(9–10): 67–95.

Anderson, M. A. (2010). Neural reuse: a fundamental organizational principle of the brain. *Behavioral and Brain Science 33*(4): 245–266.

Atmanspacher, H. (1992). Categoreal and acategoreal representation of knowledge. *Cognitive Systems 3*: 259–288.

Atmanspacher, H. (2012). Dual-aspect monism à la Pauli and Jung. *Journal of Consciousness Studies 19*(9): 96–120.

Atmanspacher, H. (2014). 20th-century versions of dual-aspect thinking. *Mind and Matter 12*: 245–288.

Atmanspacher, H. (2017). Contextual emergence in decompositional dual-aspect monism. *Mind and Matter 15*(1): 111–129.

Atmanspacher, H. and Fach, W. (2005). Acategoriality as mental instability. *Journal of Mind and Behavior 26*: 181–206.

Atmanspacher, H. and Fach, W. (2013). A structural-phenomenological typology of mind-matter correlations. *Journal of Analytical Psychology 58*: 219–244.

Atmanspacher, H. and Fach, W. (2019). Exceptional experiences of stable and unstable mental states, understood from a dual-aspect point of view. *Philosophies 4*(1): 7.

Atmanspacher, H. and Fuchs, C. A. (Eds.) (2014). *The Pauli-Jung Conjecture and Its Impact Today*. Exeter: Imprint Academic.

Atmanspacher, H. and Kronz, F. (1999). Relative onticity. In H. Atmanspacher, A. Amann and U. Müller-Herold (Eds.), *On Quanta, Mind, and Matter. Hans Primas in Context*, 273–294. Dordrecht: Kluwer.

Atmanspacher, H. and Primas, H. (2003). Epistemic and ontic quantum realities. In L. Castell and O. Ischebeck (Eds.), *Time, Quantum, Information*, 301–321. Berlin: Springer.

Atmanspacher, H., Primas, H., and Wertenschlag-Birkäuser, E. (Eds.) (1995). *Der Pauli-Jung-Dialog und seine Bedeutung für die moderne Wissenschaft.* Berlin: Springer.

Bagger, M. (2007). *The Uses of Paradox.* New York: Columbia University Press.

Bishop, R. C. and Atmanspacher, H. (2011). The causal closure of physics and free will. In R. Kane (Ed.), *Oxford Handbook of Free Will*, 101–114. Oxford: Oxford University Press.

Chalmers, D. (1996). *The Conscious Mind.* Oxford: Oxford University Press.

Deleuze, G. (1994). *Difference and Repetition.* New York: Columbia University Press.

Deleuze, G. (1999). *Expressionism in Philosophy: Spinoza.* New York: Zone Books.

Fach, W., Atmanspacher, H., Landolt, K., Wyss, T., and Rössler, W. (2013). A comparative study of exceptional experiences of clients seeking advice and of subjects in an ordinary population. *Frontiers in Psychology* 4(65): 1–10.

Fach, W. (2011). Phenomenological aspects of complementarity and entanglement in exceptional human experiences (ExE). *Axiomathes* 21(2): 233–247.

Fach, W. (2020). *Das Spektrum des Aussergewöhnlichen. Konzeptionelle Ansätze, empirisch-phänomenologische Untersuchungen und plananalytische Fallstudien zur mentalen Repräsentation bei aussergewöhnlichen Erfahrungen.* PhD thesis, University of Bern.

Feil, D. and Atmanspacher, H. (2010). Acategorial states in a representational theory of mental processes. *Journal of Consciousness Studies* 17(5/6): 72–104.

Gebser, J. (1986). *The Ever-Present Origin.* Athens, OH: Ohio University Press.

Gunther, Y. H., (Ed.) (2003). *Essays on Nonconceptual Content.* Cambridge, MA: MIT Press.

Jung, C. G. (1953). The relations between the ego and the unconscious. In *The Collected Works of C. G. Jung* (Sir H. Read, M. Fordham, and G. Adler, Eds.; W. McGuire, Exec. Ed.; R. F. C. Hull, Trans.) [hereafter *Collected Works*], Vol. 7, *Two Essays on Analytical Psychology*, 121–241. Princeton, NJ: Princeton University Press.

Jung, C. G. (1969). On the nature of the psyche. In *Collected Works*, Vol. 8, *The Structure and Dynamics of the Psyche*, 2nd ed.,159–234. Princeton, NJ: Princeton University Press.

Jung, C. G. (1970). *Collected Works,* Vol. 14, *Mysterium Coniunctionis: An Inquiry into the Separation and Synthesis of Psychic Opposites in Alchemy,* 2nd ed. Princeton, NJ: Princeton University Press.

Jung, C. G. (1972). *Synchronicity: An Acausal Connecting Principle.* London: Routledge & Kegan Paul.

Jung, C. G. and Pauli, W. (1955). *The Interpretation of Nature and the Psyche* (R. F. C. Hull and P. Silz, Trans.). New York: Pantheon.

Kapur, S. (2003). Psychosis as a state of aberrant salience: a framework linking biology, phenomenology, and pharmacology in schizophrenia. *American Journal of Psychiatry 160*: 13–23.

Kerslake, C. (2002). The vertigo of philosophy: Deleuze and the problem of immanence. *Radical Philosophy 113*. Accessible at www.generation-online. org/p/fpdeleuze8.htm.

Kerslake, C. (2007). *Deleuze and the Unconscious.* London: Continuum

Lowe, E. J. (2000). Causal closure principles and emergentism. *Philosophy 75*: 571–586.

Marshall, P. (2005). *Mystical Encounters with the Natural World.* Oxford: Oxford University Press.

Metzinger, T. (2005). Out-of-body experiences as the origin of the concept of a soul. *Mind and Matter 3*: 57–74.

Miller, C. L. (2013). Cusanus, Nicolaus. In E. N. Zalta (Ed.), *Stanford Encyclopedia of Philosophy*. Accessible at https://plato.stanford.edu/entries/cusanus/.

Montero, B. (2003). Varieties of causal closure. In S. Walter and H.-D. Heckmann (Eds.), *Physicalism and Mental Causation*, 173–187. Exeter: Imprint Academic.

Murphy, T. S. (1998). Quantum ontology: a virtual mechanics of becoming. In E. Kaufman and K. J. Heller (Eds.), *Deleuze and Guattari. New Mappings in Politics, Philosophy, and Culture*, 211–229. Minneapolis, MN: University of Minnesota Press.

Oizumi, M., Albantakis, L., and Tononi, G. (2014). From the phenomenology to the mechanisms of consciousness: integrated information theory 3.0. *PLoS Computational Biology 10*(5): e1003588.

Papineau, D. (2015). Naturalism. In E. N. Zalta (Ed.), *Stanford Encyclopedia of Philosophy*. Accessible at https://plato.stanford.edu/entries/naturalism/.

Pauli, W. (1948). Moderne Beispiele zur Hintergrundsphysik. In C. A. Meier (Ed.), *Wolfgang Pauli und C. G. Jung: Ein Briefwechsel*, 176–192. Berlin: Springer.

Stace, W. T. (1960). *Mysticism and Philosophy*. Philadelphia, PA: Lippincott.

Stubenberg, L. (2010). Neutral monism. In E. N. Zalta (Ed.), *Stanford Encyclopedia of Philosophy*. Accessible at https://plato.stanford.edu/entries/neutral-monism/.

Tononi, G. (2015). Integrated information theory. *Scholarpedia 10*(1): 4164. Accessible at http://dx.doi.org/10.4249/scholarpedia.4164.

Tononi, G., Boly, M., Massimini, M., and Koch, C. (2016). Integrated information theory: from consciousness to its physical substrate. *Nature Reviews Neuroscience 17*: 450–461.

von Meyenn, K. (Ed.) (1993). *Wolfgang Pauli: Wissenschaftlicher Briefwechsel, Band III: 1940–1949*. Berlin: Springer.

von Meyenn, K. (Ed.) (1996). *Wolfgang Pauli: Wissenschaftlicher Briefwechsel, Band IV, Teil I: 1950–1952*. Berlin: Springer.

von Meyenn, K. (Ed.) (1999). *Wolfgang Pauli: Wissenschaftlicher Briefwechsel, Band IV, Teil II: 1953–1954*. Berlin: Springer.

Chapter 7

Holistic enchantment and eternal recurrence

Anaxagoras, Nietzsche, Deleuze, Klages, and Jung on the beauty of it all

Paul Bishop

> Anaxagoras answered a man who was [...] asking why one should choose rather to be born than not by saying 'for the sake of viewing the heavens and the whole order of the universe'.
>
> (Aristotle, *Eudemian Ethics*, book 1, §5: 1216a 11–14)

In his famous encomium of Goethe in *Twilight of the Idols*, Nietzsche set out in detail exactly why he regarded this great author of German classicism so highly:

> No mere German event, but a European event; a grand attempt to surmount the eighteenth century, by a return to nature, by an *ascension* to the naturalness of the Renaissance, a kind of self-surmounting on the part of that century. — He possessed its strongest instincts: its sentimentality, its nature worship, its tendencies anti-historic, idealistic, unreal, and revolutionary (the last is only a form of the unreal). He called to his aid history, science, antiquity, and likewise Spinoza, but above all practical activity; he encircled himself with nothing but defined horizons; he did not sever himself from life, but placed himself in it; he was not desponding, and took as much as possible on himself, over himself, and into himself. What he aspired to was *totality* [...].[1]

Or to put it another way, Nietzsche regarded Goethe as an exemplar of *holism*.

For Nietzsche, the world is both disenchanted and enchanted: from a transcendental perspective (associated with Judeo-Christianity), the world is disenchanted, it is 'the work of a suffering and tormented

God',[2] and at one point even Zarathustra cries out, 'There is much filth in the world!' (*Es gibt in der Welt viel Kot*).[3] However, Zarathustra also goes on to say, 'But the world itself is not yet a filthy monster on that account', and from an immanent perspective the world is in fact enchanted — or potentially so. The means by which Nietzsche proposes to re-enchant (or rediscover the primordial enchantment of) the world is the doctrine of the eternal recurrence.

Various sources have been suggested for Nietzsche's doctrine of eternal recurrence, including Heraclitus,[4] and one of the earliest editors of Nietzsche's works, Rudolf Steiner, believed that he had discovered various sources of Nietzsche's thinking in his library — in this case, in the works of the German positivist philosopher and economist, Eugen Dühring (1833–1921):

A penetrating conception of Nietzsche's final creative period shone clearly before me as I read his marginal comments on Eugen Dühring's chief philosophical work. Dühring there develops the thought that one can conceive the cosmos at a single moment as a combination of elementary parts. Thus the history of the world would be the series of all such possible combinations. When once these should have been formed, then the first would have to return, and the whole series would be repeated. If anything thus exists in reality, it must have occurred innumerable times in the past, and must occur again innumerable times in future. Thus we should arrive at the conception of the eternal repetition of similar states of the cosmos. Dühring rejects this thought as an impossibility. Nietzsche reads this; he receives from it an impression, which works further in the depths of his soul and finally takes form within him as 'the return of the similar', which, together with the idea of the 'superman', dominates his final creative period.

I was profoundly impressed — indeed, shocked — by the impression which I received from thus following Nietzsche in his reading. For I saw what an opposition there was between the character of Nietzsche's spirit and that of his contemporaries. Dühring, the extreme positivist, who rejects everything which is not the result of a system of reasoning directed with cold and mathematical regularity, considers 'the eternal repetition of the similar' as an absurdity, and sets up the idea only to show its impossibility; but Nietzsche must take this up as his solution of the world-riddle, as an intuition arising from the depths of his own soul.[5]

Steiner emphasizes the psychological impact that this doctrine had on him, and thereby illustrates the formative intention underlying Nietzsche's formulation of the doctrine:[6]

Nietzsche's ideas of the 'eternal repetition' and of 'superman' remained long in my mind. [...] Nietzsche perceived the evolution of humanity in such a way that whatever happened at any moment has already happened innumerable times in precisely the same form, and will happen again innumerable times in future. The atomistic conception of the cosmos makes the present moment seem a certain definite combination of the smallest entities; this must be followed by another, and this in turn by yet another — until, when all possible combinations have been formed, the first must again appear. A human life with all its individual details has been present innumerable times; it will return with all its details innumerable times.

The 'repeated earth-lives' of humanity shone darkly in Nietzsche's subconsciousness. [...][7]

In one of the models of 'eternal recurrence' found in Nietzsche's *Nachlass*, he speaks of 'the great dice game of existence',[8] and another — and highly charismatic — presentation of the doctrine can be found in *Thus Spoke Zarathustra*. Following the initial presentation of the doctrine of eternal recurrence in *The Gay Science*, §341, and in *Thus Spoke Zarathustra*, Part Three, 'Of the Vision and the Riddle', in the later chapter of Part Three entitled 'The Convalescent', Zarathustra's animals proclaim him to be 'the teacher of the eternal recurrence', and they summarize this teaching for him in these words:

'I shall return, with this sun, with this eagle, with this serpent — *not* to a new life or a better life or a similar life:

I shall return eternally to this identical and self-same life, in the greatest of things and in the smallest, to teach once more the eternal recurrence of all things,

To speak once more the teaching of the great noontide of earth and man, to tell man of the Superman once more'.[9]

But are Zarathustra's animals right?

Numerous thinkers have explored the implications of the doctrine of eternal recurrence, including Lou Andreas-Salomé, Oskar Ewald, Georg Simmel, Ernst Bertram, Charles Andler, Ludwig Klages, Alfred Baeumler, Erika Emmerich, Thierry Maulnier, Karl Jaspers, Ludwig Griesz, and Martin Heidegger — as Karl Löwith (1897–1973) pointed out in his study, *Nietzsche's Philosophy of the Eternal Recurrence of the Same* (1935).[10] And to this list of names one could also add Pierre Klossowski,[11] Gilles Deleuze, and other French interpreters of Nietzsche.

Heidegger places a reading of the chapter entitled 'The Convalescent' at the centre of his essay 'Who is Nietzsche's Zarathustra?'[12] In order to answer this question, Heidegger turns to the chapter entitled 'The Convalescent' and foregrounds the passage where Zarathustra identifies himself as 'the advocate of life, the advocate of suffering, the advocate of the circle'.[13] On Heidegger's account, all three things point to the doctrine of the eternal recurrence, and he reformulates Zarathustra's answer as follows: 'Zarathustra is the teacher of the Eternal Recurrence of the same and the teacher of the Superman', adding that 'Zarathustra teaches the Superman *because* he is the teacher of the Eternal Recurrence' — and vice versa.[14]

Thus Heidegger argues that 'both doctrines', that is, eternal recurrence and the *Übermensch*, 'belong together in a circle', and 'by its circling, the doctrine accords with what is, with the circle that constitutes the Being of beings — that is, the permanent within Becoming'.[15] For Heidegger, eternal recurrence of the same is 'the name of the Being of beings', and the *Übermensch* is 'the name of the human being who corresponds to this Being'.[16]

Yet Heidegger remains concerned about the doctrine of the eternal recurrence of the same, on which he appends a note to his essay. Here he announces that Nietzsche himself knew that what Zarathustra calls his 'most abysmal thought' remains 'an enigma', and he adds that we ourselves are 'all the less free to think that we can solve the enigma' — and yet: 'the obscurity of this final thought in Western metaphysics should not seduce us into avoiding that thought by subterfuge'.[17] According to Heidegger, there are two possible kinds of subterfuge or ways of avoiding the thought of eternal recurrence. First, we can say that Nietzsche's thought eternal recurrence is 'a kind of "mysticism" and has no place before thought'; and second, we can say that 'this thought is already ancient', by identifying it with other cyclical views of the course of the world (such as the one found in Heraclitus). In Heidegger's view, neither strategy is satisfactory, and he goes on to reject the suggestion that Nietzsche's doctrine of eternal recurrence should be interpreted 'in a mechanical sense'; rather, he argues, it hints at something metaphysical — and at something beyond metaphysics:

> That Nietzsche experienced and expounded his most abysmal thought from the Dionysian standpoint only suggests that he was still compelled to think it metaphysically, and only metaphysically. But it does not preclude that this most abysmal thought conceals something unthought, which also is impenetrable to metaphysical thinking.[18]

For different reasons, albeit ones that are, as in Heidegger, indexed to Platonism and to the overcoming or overturning of Platonism — Nietzsche talks about 'inverted Platonism', while Deleuze's work has been described as an 'overturning of Platonism',[19] — Deleuze is intrigued by Nietzsche's doctrine of eternal recurrence, which he discusses at various points in his work, including in *Nietzsche and Philosophy* (1962), in *Nietzsche* (1965), and in *Difference and Repetition* (1968).[20]

In *Nietzsche and Philosophy*, for instance, Deleuze offers a reading of eternal recurrence that is at variance from that of the majority of other commentators. As it is presented in 'The Convalescent' — 'all things recur eternally, and we ourselves with them [...]', etc. — eternal recurrence involves the *identity* of what recurs. For Deleuze, however, eternal recurrence involves *similarity* and *dissimilarity*, or more precisely it is the recurrence of *dissimilarity*. According to Deleuze:

> We misinterpret the expression 'eternal return' if we understand it as 'return of the same'. It is not being that returns but rather the returning itself that constitutes being insofar as it is affirmed of

becoming, and of that which passes. It is not some one thing which returns but rather returning itself is the one thing which is affirmed of diversity or multiplicity. In other words, *identity in eternal return does not describe the nature of that which returns but*, on the contrary, *the fact of returning for that which differs*.[21]

In his 1965 study of *Nietzsche*, Deleuze reaffirms that one should avoid 'turning the Eternal Recurrence into *a return of the Same*', and he describes it as erroneous to believe that eternal recurrence refers to 'a cycle, or a return of the Same, or a return to the same' (adding it is equally erroneous to believe it refers to an ancient idea borrowed from the Greeks, the Hindus, or the Babylonians...).[22] In *Difference and Repetition*, a kind of extended gloss on ideas originally explored in relation to eternal recurrence, Deleuze declares:

> *It is not the same which returns, it is not the similar which returns*; rather, the Same is the returning of that which returns, — *in other words, of the Different*; the similar is the returning of that which returns, — *in other words, of the Dissimilar*. The repetition in the eternal return is the same, but the same in so far as it is said uniquely of difference and the different. This is a complete reversal of the world of representation, and of the sense that 'identical' and 'similar' had in that world.[23]

Rather, Deleuze prefers to read Nietzsche in terms of active and reactive forces, as several passages from *Nietzsche and Philosophy* will confirm, and the starting-point for this approach is a twofold one: first, Spinoza's observation in his *Ethics* (part 3, proposition 2, scholium) that 'no one has yet determined what the body can do';[24] and second, Nietzsche's remark that 'we are in the phase of modesty of consciousness'.[25] Although Deleuze offers what seems like a curiously abstract definition of the body as '[a] relation between dominating and dominated forces [...] whether chemical, biological, social, or political',[26] the key distinction for Deleuze is between 'superior and dominating forces' and 'inferior or dominated forces', i.e., between *active* and *reactive* forces. On this basis, Deleuze proposes the following reading of eternal recurrence:

The eternal return produces becoming-active. It is sufficient to relate the will to nothingness to the eternal return in order to realize that reactive forces do not return. However far they go, however deep the becoming-reactive of forces, reactive forces will not return. The small, petty, reactive man will not return.[27]

And in his 1965 study of Nietzsche, Deleuze is even clearer in his emphasis on the positive aspects of eternal recurrence:

Affirmation alone returns, this that can be affirmed alone returns, joy alone returns. Everything that can be denied, everything that is negation, is expelled due to the very movement of the eternal return. We were entitled to dread that the combinations of nihilism and reactivity would eternally return too. The eternal return must be compared to a wheel; yet, the movement of the wheel is endowed with centrifugal powers that drive away the entire negative. Because Being imposes itself on becoming, it expels from itself everything that contradicts affirmation, all forms of nihilism and reactivity: bad conscience, ressentiment..., we shall witness them only once. [...] The eternal return is the Repetition; but it is the Repetition that selects, the Repetition that saves. Here is the marvelous secret of a liberating and selective repetition.[28]

Yet Deleuze's reading can be challenged, not least because it appears to overlook Zarathustra's distress precisely that 'alas, man recurs eternally! The little man recurs eternally!',[29] and Deleuze's account has most recently been challenged by Michel Onfray. For as Onfray points out, to interpret the eternal return as a selective principle occludes its function as a *tragic principle* which invokes what Nietzsche elsewhere calls *amor fati* and serves as the keystone to the entire existential edifice constructed by him.[30]

An intriguing critique of Nietzsche's doctrine of eternal recurrence was advanced by a thinker who is, today, comparatively unknown but who was, in fact, one of the earliest significant commentators on Nietzsche's work, Ludwig Klages (1872–1956).[31] (Recent work on this controversial figure includes studies by Nitzan Lebovic, who has sought to situate him in the content of a so-called 'Nazi biopolitics';[32]

and Jason Ā. Josephson-Storm, who has placed Klages in a tradition that expounds the 'myth' of disenchantment, and presented him as a combination of the Derridean critique of logocentrism, the Frankfurt School critique of the Enlightenment, and the Heideggerian suspicion of technology — albeit as a 'monstrous' one, and explicitly *not* in an attempt to rehabilitate Klages.)[33]

Now in some ways Klages can be seen as an holistic thinker, inasmuch as he offers a total interpretation of reality using such concepts as spirit (*Geist*) and soul (*Seele*); in other ways he is an anti-holistic thinker, inasmuch as he conceives of reality as being radically fissured, broken, split between *Geist* and *Seele*, regarding these two forces as being radically opposed. For his 'signature concept' of spirit or *Geist*, Klages is profoundly indebted to Aristotle who, in his treatise *On the Generation of Animals*, advanced the view that, in conception, the female contributes the matter of the future composite, while the male contributes the soul. The intellect, however, enters the individual at another point: it is, in Aristotle's phrase, an 'intellect from without' (*nous thurathen*).[34] Klages himself specifically mentions this doctrine on two occasions in his main work, *The Spirit as Adversary of the Soul* (1929–1932), referring to it as 'the doctrine that the spirit is added to life from outside (= *thurathen*, according to Aristotle's expression)'.[35]

In his early treatise *Of Cosmogonic Eros* (1922;²1926) Klages stated his core thesis as follows:

> The cosmos is alive, and all life is polarized into soul (*psyche*) and body (*soma*). Wherever there is living body, there is soul; wherever soul, there is living body. The soul is the sense of the body, the image of the body is the appearance of the soul. Whatever appears, that has a sense; and every sense reveals itself as it appears. Sense [*der Sinn*] is experienced internally, appearance [*die Erscheinung*] externally. The former must become image if it is to be communicated, and the image must become internal again, for it to have an effect. Those are, expressed without metaphor, the poles of reality.[36]

What Klages presents to us here in 'cosmic' terms — a dialectical interrelation between dynamic opposites, a union born of an energic tension — is, he thinks in *The Spirit as Adversary of the Soul*, also observable in world history:

> The history of humanity shows us in humankind and *only* in humankind the war 'to the knife' between all-embracing life and a power *outside space and time*, which wants to sever the poles and thereby destroy them, to 'de-soul' the body, disembody the soul: it is called spirit [*Geist*] (Logos, Pneuma, Nous).[37]

And in book 4, part 3, chapter 54, Klages offers the following remarkable image to describe his thesis:

> The spirit resembles a wedge driven into the life-cell, a wedge whose goal is to tear it in half or, less metaphorically expressed, to deprive the body of soul, to deprive the soul of body, and in this way to kill life itself.[38]

So it would be fair to say that Klages's central thesis is admirably summed up in the title of his major work: for him, *Geist* is the enemy of *Seele*, or (more usually) 'the spirit is the adversary of the soul', or (less conventionally) 'mind is the opponent of psyche'. Klages would have us believe that the rational mind has split us apart from the passionate-intuitive part of our selves, so that our (instrumental) consciousness is purchased at the price of alienation from the emotional and affective component of our identity.

In his book-length survey of Nietzsche's philosophy published in 1926 and entitled *The Psychological Achievements of Friedrich Nietzsche* (*Die psychologischen Errungenschaften Friedrich Nietzsches*), Klages examined Nietzsche's philosophical 'research goals' and 'methods', before considering the 'applications and results' of this investigative methodology and discussing a number of key ideas and motifs in Nietzsche's philosophy.[39] In the third part of this study, Klages offers a wide-ranging critique of Nietzsche, beginning with what he calls Nietzsche's 'Socratism', by which Klages means — in this respect, anticipating Heidegger's later critique in his Nietzsche lectures —[40] that Nietzsche failed to escape the discursive space of Platonic (i.e., metaphysical) thought as found in the dialogues attributed to Socrates.

Moreover, as far as Klages is concerned, the doctrine of eternal recurrence is a nonsensical idea and one of Nietzsche's biggest mistakes; in Klages's eyes, it was conceptually flawed through and through:

> Think about it: a Heraclitean as convinced as Nietzsche was knows no things, therefore no similarity of things, therefore no *repetition* of any kind. Similar things can recur, identical things never. Conversely, the assumption of repetitions constitutes the defining characteristic of mechanistic thought, irrespective of whether one is thinking of the numbers of plates that are manufactured from one and the same factory model, or the rotations of a wheel at a certain speed, *or* for that matter a *cosmic* wheel, whose each and every rotation requires billion upon billions of years. So much is evident. Simply unceasing repetition, the symbol of all mechanistic thought and the most unconditional counterexpression of life, is affirmed by Nietzsche the Heraclitean and in *The Will to Power*, where he tries to cover up the contradiction by separating the *infinity* of the repetitions from a merely *finite* world machine of mechanistics through an emphasis on its terrible prospect: the most extreme exaggeration of a baroque ideal called perpetuum mobile![41]

In order to appreciate this critique of Nietzsche, we have to see it in the context of Klages's philosophy as a whole, in which two ideas are central. First, there is the doctrine of the 'reality of images' (*die Wirklichleit der Bilder*), an astonishing attempt on the part of Klages to reverse the entire Western philosophical tradition and argue for the ontological superiority of the *image* as opposed to the *thing* (materialism) or the *Idea* (Platonic idealism).[42]

On the account of the doctrine of the 'reality of images' offered by Franz Tenigl,[43] these images are powers or essences of the soul that are the basis of all cosmic (elementary) or cellular (organic) phenomena. In such organisms as flowers, plants, or human beings, they manifest themselves and shape matter in the form of growth, metabolism, and inheritance. In animals they additionally awaken drives and instincts that initiate motions. In human beings, too, these vegetative and animal vital processes manifest themselves, while over and beyond these there arises, independent of the drives, the 'capacity for vision'. In this way the world itself awakens and reveals itself for human beings to be a reality of images, thus enabling them to create symbols of reality that in turn renews for all intuitively envisioned individuals the revelation of essences. Here lies the root of myth, religious cult, and festival, as well as poetry and art.

Although these powers of the soul are invisible, they are called 'images' because they can appear to humans and to animals alike in sensorily intuitable images. Every intuitive image (*Anschauungsbild*), which is split up across different senses, is governed by a meaning or a significance with which the essence, the power of the soul, manifests itself. The experiential process constitutes a polaristic relation between the images of the world as they manifest themselves (the macrocosm) and the receptive soul (the microcosm). This means that it is only because an essential life appears in the images that we feel or experience ourselves as being alive.

Klages himself defined his doctrine of the reality of images in the following terms:

> The reality of images is a reality of appearance [*eine Wirklichkeit der Erscheinung*] insofar as it is a reality of souls that appear or, since souls are at any rate alive, a reality of constantly changing *life*. The comparison: real, more real, most real means: alive, more alive, most alive, and the basis for all gradations of value appropriate to the world lies in the degree of *vital fullness* [*Lebensfülle*].[44]

The 'reality of images' is a reality that 'reaches back in an endless chain into what has no beginning' (*endlos verkettet zurückreicht ins Anbeginnlose*), for 'primordial images are souls of the past as they appear' (*Urbilder sind erscheinende Vergangenheitsseelen*);[45] time and again Klages emphasizes that these 'images' (*Bilder*) are 'powers that manifest themselves' (*wirkende Mächte*).[46] For Klages, 'reality' is 'pure happening' (*Geschehen schlechthin*)[47] —or in Deleuzian terms, an 'event'.

Second, and related to the doctrine of the reality of images, is Klages's notion of *elementare Ähnlichkeit* or 'elementary similarity'.

> If somebody looks without inhibition at an object and its reflection, he or she judges the appearances of both as being completely

equal (in spite of the fact that in the mirror-image right and left are of course reversed). How much more closely by contrast must we determine the relation of the fleeting images of primordial space to each and every present impression-image [*Eindrucksbild*] of sensory space, since here being equal certainly does not prevail? Our answer is as follows: both are connected by means of *elementary similarity*.[48]

The notion of 'elementary similarity' is the means by which Klages explains that reality as we experience it is intuited as a coherent whole.[49] In each sensory impression (*Eindruck*) the temporal-spatial images converge because of their 'similarity' or, as Klages puts it: first, 'impression images [*Eindrucksbilder*] emerge' — literally, 'coagulate' — 'from the concurrently experienced similarities of perceived primordial images'; and second, 'the meaningful grouping of the impression images results in accordance with elementary similarities'.[50] On this conception of the 'reality of life' (*Wirklichkeit des Lebens*) everything is connected, not by cause and effect, but exclusively according to 'elementary similarities', so that 'the weaving power of all that *belongs* together through relation or opposition' is located in 'the workings of essences [...] which appear in intuitive images' (*Wirksamkeit von Wesen ... die in den Anschauungsbildern erscheinen*).[51] Or to put it another way, 'if neither spatial and temporal continuity nor qualities would, without concurrently experienced similarities, be perceptible, then it is clear that the conditions for similarities must be present for it to be possible for them to appear'.[52] In *Handwriting and Character*, Klages argues that reproduction is the recurrence of similar images across similar intervals of time,[53] and even the movement of individual beings derives from elementary similarity,[54] so that it is no exaggeration to say that 'the means of all real self-realization [*alles wirklichen Wirkens*] is elementary similarity'.[55]

Playing on the etymology of the word 'symbol' — from σύμβολον (symbolon), cf. συμβάλλειν (symballein), i.e., 'to throw together' — Klages declares that 'the symbol-discovering act does *not* separate everything and instead embraces in one that which on the level of objective thought would disintegrate into what is experienced and experience itself, object and subject, world and ego, there and here, once upon a time and now',[56] for in symbolic thought everything belongs together. Instead of differentiating and making distinctions, what comes to the fore is elementary similarity, and out of this elementary similarity arises a *symbolic world*. In a lengthy footnote added to his discussion of Romanticism in chapter 57 of *The Spirit as Adversary of the Soul*, Klages observes:

> Just as relations can be established between all concepts, so connections can be demonstrated between all symbols, and just as all concepts are different from each other, so no symbol is identical in meaning to another. The content of the circle symbol is one thing if the circle is thought of as rotating, and another when the circle is motionless.[57]

According to Klages, the notion of *identity* informs the kind of perception he associates with *der Geist*, i.e., with spirit, mind, or intellect; and, for Klages, this *Geist* is an essentially negative agent. (This position has earned him the reputation of being an irrationalist, although — as one can see from the intricacy of his argumentation — this is far from being the case.) By contrast, the notion of similarity informs the kind of perception he associates with *die Seele*, i.e., with the soul or the psyche, and which he regards as essentially *symbolic*:

> We have repeatedly given examples of the belief in images of prehistory and *its* reflective form of non-conceptual, but symbolic thought. Now we want to arrange — from the miraculous tales and liturgies, from the reverence for fetishes and magical beings, from soothsaying and superstitions, from sacred customs and celebrations, restrictions and commands, or in short from the entire heritage of prehistorical humankind in a particular series — a greater range of witnesses to demonstrate that the life-bound spirit, despite the limitless diversity of its creations and no less in its degenerate and disintegrating as in its healthy and perfect ones, is based on the rule of the belief in images over the belief in the reality of things and in all expressions without exception the efficacy (even if by no means a discursive consciousness) allows one to discern the following fundamental thought: the essential unity of images themselves with the active powers of the world, of the images among themselves according to the extent of their elementary similarity, and of a special image with its symbolic signs,

and then again of the image-receiving and the sign-giving soul of humankind.[58]

To put it another way, Klages is exploring a form of non-identity thinking he calls *symbolic*, and in this respect there is a significant point of contact with C.G. Jung, another twentieth-century thinker who is interested in the symbol. (In twentieth-century thinking it is possible to discern two major lines of thought: those who are primarily interested in signs, from Saussure through to such structuralists and post-structuralists as Derrida, Foucault, Lacan, and Deleuze, and another — in some respects, more neglected or more subterranean tradition — that is interested in symbols, from J. J. Bachofen through to Cassirer, Klages, and Jung.)

Underpinning the idea of the symbol is the concept of *homology*, related to the notion of *homoiōsis*,[59] a doctrine that goes back to the pre-Socratic philosopher Anaxagoras of Clazomenae, an important intellectual source for Klages.[60] For reasons of space, we cannot explore Anaxagoras's teaching (as it has come down us in fragmentary form) in detail here,[61] but its significance was rightly appreciated by Nietzsche. (For his part, Heidegger seems to have been more interested in Anaximander, Heraclitus, or Parmenides than in Anaxagoras.)[62] Nietzsche discussed the thought of Anaxagoras in its intellectual-historic context of pre-Socratic thought in *Philosophy in the Tragic Age of the Greeks* (1872–1873) and in his lecture course on *The Pre-Platonic Philosophers* (first given in 1869–1870).[63] In the first of these works, he summarized the achievement of Anaxagoras as residing in his conception of *nous*:

> The Spirit [*nous*] of Anaxagoras is a creative artist. It is, in fact, the most tremendous mechanical and architectural genius, creating with the simplest means the most impressive forms and orbits, creating a movable architecture, as it were, but ever from the irrational free random choosing that lies in the artist's depths. It is as though Anaxagoras were pointing to Phidias and — confronted by the enormous art object of the cosmos — were proclaiming as he would of the Parthenon, "Coming-to-be is not a moral but an aesthetic phenomenon."[64]

In effect, Nietzsche's Anaxagoras anticipates one of the central claims of *The Birth of Tragedy*, that is, that 'the world is justified as an *aesthetic* phenomenon'.[65] And in a footnote to his notes for his lectures, Nietzsche outlined the core idea of Anaxagoras as follows:

> A substitute for religion in the circles of the educated. Philosophy as an esoteric cult of the man of knowledge in contrast to folk religion. Mind [νοῦς] as the architect and artist, like Phidias. The majesty of simple, unmoved beauty — Pericles as orator. The simplest possible means. Many beings [ὄντα], countless many. Nothing goes lost. Dualism of motion. The entire Mind [νοῦς] moves. Against Parmenides: he accounts the senses, the will to *nous*, but he must now carry out a new distinction, that of vegetative and animal.[66]

In one of his surviving fragments, Anaxagoras proposes the quasi-atomistic theory that the universe is composed of the 'seeds of all things' (DK 59 B4), and according to Aristotle, these 'seeds of all things' are described as *homoiomeries*, that is, things that are homogeneous components.[67]

The term *homoiomeries* and the notion of *homoiōsis* can also be found in Plato; for instance, in the notion of *homoiōsis theōi* = 'likeness to God' as in the remark made by Socrates to Theodorus in the *Theaetetus* (176a–b), 'Therefore we ought to try to escape from earth to the dwelling of the gods as quickly as we can; and to escape is to become like God, so far as this is possible; and to become like God is to become righteous and holy and wise'.[68] This notion of *homoiōsis theōi* as the end (*telos*) of life which is to be attained by knowledge (*gnōsis*) is maintained by Iamblichus (*Protrepticus*, chap. 3) where he writes: 'Knowledge of the gods is virtue and wisdom and perfect happiness, and makes us like to the gods'.[69] This Neoplatonic tradition continues down to the thirteenth century where, in *De visione beatifica* and *De intellectu et intelligibili*, Dietrich von Freiberg drew (as did Meister Eckhart) a distinction between *similitudo Dei* and *imago Dei*, the former being for the created order and the latter applicable for the intellect.[70]

The notion of homology or homoiōsis underpins the symbol, which for its operational efficacy relies on a likeness or similarity between itself and what it symbolizes. As Klages points out, alluding to the declaration made by Plotinus in his *Ennead* entitled 'On Beauty' (I.6.9), 'For one must come to the sight with a seeing power made akin and like to what is seen. No eye ever saw the sun without becoming sun-like [...]',[71] these words 'inspired those much admired verses by Goethe':[72]

> If the eye were not sunny,
> How could we perceive light?
> [*Wär' nicht das Auge sonnenhaft*
> *Die Sonne könnt es nie erblicken?*][73]

On the one hand, this saying confirms the thesis (found in Homer, Parmenides, and Empedocles) that only like can recognize like (the so-called *homoion* theory),[74] and Klages identifies this position held by Anaxagoras and his notion of *homoiomeries*.[75]

For Klages this tradition continues into the Renaissance, in the form of Francesco Patrizzi's maxim that cognition means to become one with the object (*cognitio nihil est aliud, quam Coitio quaedam cum suo cognobili*),[76] and Tommaso Campenella's definition of the act of knowledge as a fusing with the object (*cognoscere est fieri rem cognitam*).[77] On the other, Klages identifies the view also attributed to Anaxagoras that things are only recognized by their opposites (i.e., coldness by warmth, warmth by coldness, brightness by darkness, darkness by brightness, sweetness by bitterness, bitterness by sweetness), an intuition of 'the polar character of [...] similarity' as well as a recognition of the 'suffering quality [*Erleidniston*] of sensory experience'.[78]

Just as Klages envisages two essentially opposing powers, i.e., soul and spirit, so he posits two faculties that are related to each of them: one vital, one intellectual. In the most extreme case, this means that the spirit grasps only its productions, torn away from life (and in the sphere of Being), and hence also itself (cf. Anaxagoras, DK59 B12); life, by contrast, lives and experiences only itself, that is, what is alive and vital. It falls to the personal ego to link both worlds within itself, for only it can bear within itself both aspects and both faculties. Thus on Klages's view the tragedy of human life resides in its impulse to create a holistic sense of existence out of an ontological being that is irremediably, irredeemably fissured and broken.

* * *

Eternal recurrence is a fascinating doctrine that has intrigued thinkers as diverse as the German sociologist and political economist, Max Weber (1864–1920), who refers to it in a footnote in *The Protestant Ethic and the Spirit of Capitalism* (1905),[79] and the Russian mathematician and esotericist P. D. Ouspensky (1878–1947), who uses the idea as a motif in his novel, *Strange Life of Ivan Osokin* (1915).[80] Most recently it has been used by Anthony Peake to support his hypothesis that there is evidence for a life after death;[81] curiously enough, one of the most recent academic interpretations of *Thus Spoke Zarathustra*, Paul S. Loeb's *The Death of Nietzsche's Zarathustra* (2010), lends credence to this hypothesis by arguing that, as Zarathustra dies, he experiences on his deathbed a revelation that shows him how his life is endlessly repeating — enabling him to return to his identical life, recollect this revelation, and go beyond the human to become an *Übermensch*.[82]

In the German philosophical tradition, it attracted the attention of Herbert Marcuse, who discussed the eternal return in Aristotle, Hegel, and Nietzsche in a 'philosophical interlude' in his *Eros and Civilization: A Philosophical Inquiry into Freud* (1955),[83] where he cited the words of the animals in 'The Convalescent', 'Everything goes, everything returns; the wheel of existence rolls for ever. [...] Everything departs, everything meets again; the ring of existence is true to itself for ever. / Existence begins in every instant; the ball There rolls around every Here. The middle is everywhere. The path of eternity is crooked',[84] and he remarks on this image of the closed circle as 'the symbol of being-as-end-in-itself':

> While Aristotle reserved it to the *nous theos*, while Hegel identified it with the absolute idea, Nietzsche envisages the eternal return of the finite exactly as it is — in its full concreteness and finiteness. This is the total affirmation of the life instincts, repelling all escape and negation. The eternal return is the will and vision of an *erotic* attitude toward being for which necessity and fulfilment coincide.[85]

And it also intrigued the eclectic German-Jewish critic and essayist, Walter Benjamin (1892–1940), who wrote in his essay, 'Central Park', §35:

> Eternal recurrence is an attempt to link the two antinomic principles of happiness with one another: namely that of eternity and that of the yet once again. — The idea of eternal recurrence conjures out of the *Misère* (wretchedness) of (the) time the speculative idea (or the phantasmagoria) of happiness. Nietzsche's heroism is the counterpart of Baudelaire's which, out of the wretchedness of philistine routine, conjures up the phantasmagoria of the modern.[86]

In this sense, Benjamin comes to the conclusion that must surely count as the most devastating statement ever of disenchantment — 'That "things just go on" *is* the catastrophe'!

This idea, that 'hell [...] is not something that lies before us, but *this life here*', is one that we also find expressed by Jung in his *Red Book*. In 'The Conception of the God', Jung says:

> He who journeys to Hell also becomes Hell; therefore do not forget from whence you come. The depths are stronger than us; so do not be heroes, be clever and drop the heroics, since nothing is more dangerous than to play the hero. The depths want to keep you; they have not returned very many up to now, and therefore men fled from the depths and attacked them. What if the depths, due to the assault, now change themselves into death? But the depths indeed have changed themselves into death; therefore when they awoke they inflicted a thousandfold death. We cannot slay death, as we have already taken all life from it. If we still want to overcome death, then we must enliven it.[87]

Jung's *Red Book*, which is remarkable in so many ways, is not least remarkable for its insistence on the positivity of life, despite (or because of its) recognition of the negativity of life. As Jung put it in *Transformations and Symbols of the Libido* (1911–1912), later revised as *Symbols of Transformation* (1952):

It is hard to believe that this teeming world is too poor to provide an object for human love — it offers boundless opportunities to everyone. It is rather the inability to love which robs a person of these opportunities. The world is empty only to him who does not know how to direct his libido towards things and people, and to render them alive and beautiful. What compels us to create a substitute from within ourselves is not an external lack, but our own inability to include anything outside ourselves in our love.[88]

And thus the *Red Book*, as the imagistic (or intuitive or symbolic) source-book of Jung's later, theoretical writings on analytical psychology, also includes a positive message:

Therefore on your journey be sure to take golden cups full of the sweet drink of life, red wine, and give it to dead matter, so that it can win life back. The dead matter will change into black serpents. Do not be frightened, the serpents will immediately put out the sun of your days, and a night with wonderful will-o'-the-wisps will come over you.[89]

Notes

1 Nietzsche, *Twilight of the Idols*, 'Roving expeditions of an inopportune philosopher', §49, 'Goethe', in Nietzsche, *The Case of Wagner, Nietzsche Contra Wagner, The Twilight of the Idols; The Antichrist* [*Works*, vol. 3], tr. T. Common, London: T. Fischer Unwin, 1899, pp. 218–19.
2 Nietzsche, *Thus Spoke Zarathustra*, Part One, 'Of the afterworldsmen', in *Thus Spoke Zarathustra*, tr. R.J. Hollingdale, 1969, p. 58.
3 Nietzsche, *Thus Spoke Zarathustra*, Part Three, 'Of old and new law-tables', §14; *Zarathustra*, tr. Hollingdale, p. 222.
4 For further discussion, see J. N. Berry, 'Nietzsche and the Greeks', in K. Gemes and J. Richardson (eds), *The Oxford Handbook of Nietzsche*, Oxford: Oxford University Press, 2013, pp. 83–107 (esp. §3, 'Heraclitus', pp. 91–98); and B. Magus, 'The connection between Nietzsche's doctrine of eternal recurrence, Heraclitus, and the Stoics', *Helios*, 1976, vol. 3, 3–21.
5 R. Steiner, *The Story of My Life*, ed. H. Collinson, London; New York: Anthroposophical Publishing; Anthroposophic Press, 1928, pp. 182–83.

6 Cf. 'My philosophy brings the triumphant idea of which all other modes of thinking will ultimately perish. It is the great cultivating idea [...]' (*The Will to Power*, §1053; in Nietzsche, *The Will to Power*, ed. W. Kaufmann, tr. W. Kaufmann and R.J. Hollingdale, New York: Vintage Books, 1968, p. 544.

7 Steiner, *The Story of My Life*, p. 186.

8 *Will to Power*, §1066; *The Will to Power*, tr. Kaufmann and Hollingdale, p. 549.

9 Nietzsche, *Thus Spoke Zarathustra*, Part Three, 'The convalescent', §2; in *Zarathustra*, tr. Hollingdale, pp. 237–38.

10 K. Löwith, *Nietzsche's Philosophy of the Eternal Recurrence of the Same* [¹1935; ²1956; ³1978], tr. J. H. Lomax, Berkeley, Los Angeles, London: University of California Press, 1997, p. 196.

11 See P. Klossowski, *Nietzsche and the Vicious Circle* [1969], tr. D. W. Smith, Chicago; London: University of Chicago Press; Athlone Press, 1997.

12 Originally published as M. Heidegger, 'Wer ist Nietzsches Zarathustra?', in *Vorträge und Aufsätze*, Pfullingen: Neske, 1954, pp. 101–26; tr. by B. Magus as 'Who is Nietzsche's Zarathustra?', *The Review of Metaphysics*, 1967, vol. 20, no. 3, 411–431, and cited here from D. B. Allison (ed.), *The New Nietzsche*, Cambridge, MA, and London: MIT Press, 1985, pp. 64–79.

13 Nietzsche, *Thus Spoke Zarathustra*, 'The convalescent', §1; in *Zarathustra*, tr. Hollingdale, p. 233.

14 Heidegger, in Allison (ed.), *New Nietzsche*, p. 75.

15 Heidegger, in Allison (ed.), *New Nietzsche*, p. 75.

16 Heidegger, in Allison (ed.), p. 77. In the sense that he uses the term 'Being of beings', Heidegger is explicitly drawing on Schelling's treatise of 1809 on human freedom (cf. *New Nietzsche*, p. 79): 'In the final and highest instance there is no other Being than Will. Will is primordial Being, and all predicates apply to it alone — groundless, eternity, independence of time, self-affirmation! All philosophy strives only to find this highest expression' (F.W.J. Schelling, *Philosophical Investigation concerning the Nature of Human Freedom and its Object*, tr. J. Gutmann, La Salle, IL: Open Court, 1992, p. 24).

17 Heidegger, in Allison (ed), *New Nietzsche*, p. 78.

18 Heidegger, in Allison (ed.), *New Nietzsche*, p. 79.

19 See J. Ramey, *The Hermetic Deleuze: Philosophy and Spiritual Ordeal*, Durham and London: Duke University Press, 2012, p. 126.

20 For further discussion, see P. D'Iorio, 'The eternal return: Genesis and interpretation', *Lexicon Philosophicum: International Journal for the History of Texts and Ideas*, 2014, vol. 2, 41–96 (p. 42).

21 G. Deleuze, *Nietzsche and Philosophy* [1962], tr. H. Tomlinson, London and New York: Continuum, 2006, p. 48.

22 G. Deleuze, *Nietzsche*, Paris: PUF, 1965, pp. 36 and 41.

23 G. Deleuze, *Difference and Repetition* [1968], tr. P. Patton, London: Bloomsbury, 2014, p. 391.

24 'For indeed, no one has yet determined what the body can do, that is, experience has not yet taught anyone what the body can do from the laws of Nature alone, insofar as Nature is only considered to be corporeal, and what the body can do only if it is determined by the mind. For no one has yet come to know the structure of the body so accurately that he could explain all its functions – not to mention that many things are observed in the lower animals which far surpass human ingenuity, and that sleep-walkers do a great many things in their sleep which they would not dare to awake. This shows well enough that the body itself, simply from the laws of its own nature, can do many things which its mind wonders at' (Benedict Spinoza, *Ethics*, tr. E. Curley, in *A Spinoza Reader*, Princeton, NJ: Princeton University Press, 1994, pp. 155–156).

25 Nietzsche, *The Will to Power*, §676, 'On the origin of our evaluations'; *The Will to Power*, tr. Kaufmann and Hollingdale, p. 357.

26 Deleuze, *Nietzsche and Philosophy*, tr. Tomlinson, p. 37.

27 Deleuze, *Nietzsche and Philosophy*, tr. Tomlinson, p. 66.

28 Deleuze, *Nietzsche*, pp. 38 and 40.

29 Nietzsche, *Thus Spoke Zarathustra*, tr. Hollingdale, p. 236.

30 M. Onfray, *La Construction du surhomme* [*Contre-historie de la philosophie*, vol. 7], Paris: Grasset, 2011, p. 281. On *amor fati*, see p. 286: 'Here is the meaning of *amor fati*: to love one's destiny, to consent to it with the most total adherence, to desire it, to will it. When one loves what happens to us, one gives no quarter: what arises from what is evil, what is negative, from suffering forms part of it. There is no question of removing from what takes place what suits us by refusing and challenging what annoys us. The eternal recurrence does not select, it reiterates what has happened — including suffering'.

31 For an overview of Klages's philosophy, see P. Bishop, *Ludwig Klages and the Philosophy of Life: A Vitalist Toolkit*, London and New York: Routledge, 2018.

32 N. Lebovic, *The Philosophy of Life and Death: Ludwig Klages and the Rise of a Nazi Biopolitics*, New York: Palgrave Macmillan, 2013.

33 J. Ā. Josephson-Storm, *The Myth of Disenchantment: Magic, Modernity, and the Birth of the Human Sciences*, Chicago and London: University of Chicago Press, 2017, pp. 209–239 (pp. 213–15 and 209). My thanks to Roderick Main for bringing this work to my attention.

34 Aristotle, *De Anima (On the Soul)*, tr. H. Lawson-Tancred, 'Introduction', p. 95. See *De Generatione Animalium*, Book 2, 736 b 27 ('Reason alone enters in, as an additional factor, from outside') and 744 b 22 ('a mind, external to them') (Aristotle, *Generation of Animals*, tr. A.L. Peck, London; Cambridge, MA: Heinemann; Harvard University Press, 1943, pp. 170–71 and 230–31); cf. Aristotle, *"De Partibus Animalium" I and "De Generatione Animalium" I (with passages from II.1–3)*, tr. D.N. Balme, Oxford: Clarendon Press, 1972, pp. 63–64 and 159–60.

35 Ludwig Klages, *Der Geist als Widersacher der Seele*, 6th edn, Bonn: Bouvier, 1981, p. 369, cf. p. 868.

36 Klages, *Vom kosmogonischen Eros*, in Ludwig Klages, *Sämtliche Werke*, ed. E. Frauchinger, G. Funke, K. J. Goffmann, R. Heiss, and H. E. Schröder, 9 vols, Bonn: Bouvier, 1964–2000, vol. 3, pp. 353–497 (p. 390).

37 Klages, *Der Geist als Widersacher der Seele*, p. 390.

38 Klages, *Der Geist als Widersacher der Seele*, p. 755.

39 Ludwig Klages, *Die psychologischen Errungenschaften Friedrich Nietzsches*, Leipzig: Barth, 1926. For further discussion of Klages's relation to Nietzsche, see P. Bishop, 'Ludwig Klages's early reception of Friedrich Nietzsche', *Oxford German Studies*, 2002, vol. 31, 129–60; and 'Ein Kind Zarathustras und eine nicht-metaphysische Auslegung der ewigen Wiederkehr', in *Hestia: Jahrbuch des Klages-Gesellschaft*, 2002/2003, vol. 21, 15–37.

40 'In the thought of will to power, Nietzsche anticipates the metaphysical ground of the consummation of the modern age. In the thought of will to power, metaphysical thinking itself completes itself in advance. Nietzsche, the thinker of the thought of will to power, is the *last metaphysician* of the West. The age whose consummation unfolds in his thought, the modern age, is the final age' (M. Heidegger, *Nietzsche: Volumes 3 and 4*, vol. 3, *The Will to Power as Knowledge and as Metaphysics*, ed. D. RF. Krell, tr. J. Stambaugh, D. F. Krell, and F. A. Capuzzi, New York: HarperCollins, 1991, Part One, chapter 1, p. 8).

41 Klages, *Errungenschaften Nietzsches*, pp. 215–16.

42 For further discussion of Klages's difficult notion of the 'reality of images', see H. E. Schröder, 'Einführung in das Lebenswerk von Ludwig Klages', in Schröder (ed.), *Schiller — Nietzsche — Klages: Abhandlungen und Essays zur Geistesgeschichte der Gegenwart*, Bonn: Bouvier, 1974, pp. 269–318 (esp. pp. 281–88); H. Kasdorff, 'Die nie zu bestastende Wirklichkeit der Bilder: Ein Hinweis auf Ludwig Klages', in *Ludwig Klages: Gesammelte Aufsätze und Vorträge zu seinem Werk*, Bonn: Bouvier, 1984, pp. 170–86; and G. Böhme, 'Die Wirklichkeit der Bilder und ihr Gebrauch', *Hestia: Jahrbuch der Klages-Gesellschaft*, 2004–2007, vol. 22, 137–48.

43 F. Tenigl, 'Ludwig Klages', in *Metzler-Philosophen-Lexikon: Von den Vorsokratikern bis zu den Neuen Philosophen*, ed. B. Lutz and N. Retlich, 2nd edn, Stuttgart and Weimar: Metzler, 1995, pp. 459–63.

44 Klages, *Ausdrucksbewegung und Gestaltungskraft: Grundlegung der Wissenschaft vom Ausdruck*, in *Sämtliche Werke*, vol. 6, pp. 139–313 (p. 257).

45 Klages, *Der Geist als Widersacher der Seele*, p. 846; cf. *Vom kosmogonischen Eros*, in *Sämtliche Werke*, vol. 3, p. 470.

46 Klages, *Der Geist als Widersacher der Seele*, p. 1237.

47 Klages, *Der Geist als Widersacher der Seele*, p. 1132.

48 Klages, *Der Geist als Widersacher der Seele*, p. 346.

49 R. Müller, *Das verzwistete Ich — Ludwig Klages und sein philosophisches Hauptwerk "Der Geist als Widersacher der Seele"*, Berne and Frankfurt am Main: Lang, 1971, pp. 60–63.

50 Klages, *Der Geist als Widersacher der Seele*, p. 375.

51 Klages, *Der Geist als Widersacher der Seele*, pp. 379 and 401.

52 Klages, *Der Geist als Widersacher der Seele*, pp. 1132–33.

53 Klages, *Handschrift und Charakter: Gemeinverständlicher Abriß der graphologischen Technik*, Bonn: Bouvier, 1989, p. 36.

54 Klages, *Der Geist als Widersacher der Seele*, pp. 1047 and 1136–37.

55 Klages, *Der Geist als Widersacher der Seele*, p. 1132.

56 Klages, *Der Geist als Widersacher der Seele*, p. 1195.

57 Klages, *Der Geist als Widersacher der Seele*, p. 1444, note 20.

58 Klages, *Der Geist als Widersacher der Seele*, pp. 1257–58.

59 For a discussion of the conceptual distinction between *homology* and *analogy*, see C. Louguet, 'Anaxagore: Analogie, proportion, identité', *Philosophie antique*, 2013, vol. 13, 117–45.

60 Anaxagoras of Clazomenae, *"Fragments" and "Testimoniae": A Text and Translation with Notes and Essays*, ed. P. Curd, Toronto, Buffalo, and London: University of Toronto Press, 2007.

61 For an overview of Anaxagoras as one of the earliest proponents of holism, see P. Curd, 'Anaxagoras and the theory of everything', in P. Curd and D. W. Graham, *The Oxford Companion to Presocratic Philosophy*, Oxford and New York: Oxford University Press, 2008, pp. 230–49.

62 M. Heidegger, *Early Greek Thinking*, tr. D. F. Krell and F. A. Capuzzi, New York: HarperSanFrancisco, 1984; and M. Heidegger, *The Beginning of Western Philosophy: Interpretation of Anaximander and Parmenides*, tr. R. Rojcewicz, Bloomington, IN: Indiana University Press, 2015.

63 F. Nietzsche, *Philosophy in the Tragic Age of the Greeks*, tr. M. Cowan, Washington, DC: Regnery, 1962, §14–§19 (pp. 90–117); and *The Pre-Platonic Philosophers*, ed. and tr. G. Whitlock, Urbana, IL, and Chicago: University of Illinois Press, 2001, pp. 94–105.

64 Nietzsche, *Philosophy in the Tragic Age of the Greeks*, §19; tr. Cowan, pp. 112–13.

65 Nietzsche, *The Birth of Tragedy*, 'Attempt at a self-criticism', §5; cf. §5 and §24, in: *Basic Writings*, ed. and tr. W. Kaufmann, New York: Modern Library, 1968, pp. 22, 52 and 141.

66 Nietzsche, *The Pre-Platonic Philosophers*, p. 229 (tr. modified); cf. 'Die vorplatonischen Philosophen', in *Vorlesungsaufzeichnungen (WS 1871/72 –WS 1874/75) [Werke: Kritische Gesamtausgabe*, II. Abteilung, vol. 4], ed. F. Bornmann and M. Carpitella, Berlin and New York: de Gruyter, 1995, p. 304.

67 See *Physics*, book 3, §4, 203a19-22: 'Those who make [the elements] infinite in number, as Anaxagoras and Democritus do, say that the infinite is continous by contact — compounded of the homogeneous parts according to the one, of the seedmass of the atomic shapes according to the other' (Aristotle, *Complete Works*, ed. J. Barnes, 2 vols, Princeton, NJ: Princeton University Press, 1984, vol. 1, p. 345; *On the Heavens*, book 3, §3, 302a28-31: 'Now Anaxagoras opposes Empedocles' view of the elements... His elements are the homoeomerous things, viz. flesh, bone, and the like' (*Complete Works*, vol. 1, p. 495); *On Generation and Corruption*, book 1, §1, 314a20-21: 'Anaxagoras posits as elements the "homoeomeries", viz. bone, flesh, marrow, and everything else which is such that part and whole are synonymous' (*Complete Works*, vol. 1, p. 512); *Metaphysics*, book 1, §3, 984a12–16: 'Anaxagoras of Clazomenae [...] says the principles are infinite in number; for he says almost all things that are homogeneous are generated and destroyed (as water and fire is) only by aggregation and segregation, and are not in any other sense generated or destroyed, but remain eternally' (*Complete Works*, vol. 2, p. 1556); and *Metaphysics*, book 1, §7, 988a26–29:: 'Plato spoke of the great and the small, the Italians [i.e., the Pythagoreans, because Pythagoras founded his society at Croton] of the infinite, Empedocles of fire, earth, water, and air, Anaxagoras of the infinity of homogeneous things' (*Complete Works*, vol. 2, p. 1562).

68 Plato, *Theaetetus; Sophist* [*Works*, vol. 2], tr. H. N. Fowler, London: Heinemann; New York: Putnam, 1921, pp. 127 and 129.

69 Iamblichus, *Protrepticus*, §3; cited in A. Uždavinys (ed.), *The Golden Chain: An Anthology of Platonic and Pythagorean Philosophy*, Bloomington, IN: World Wisdom, 2004, pp. xv and 300.

70 See M. L. Führer, 'The agent intellect in the writings of Meister Dietrich of Freiberg and its influence on the Cologne School', in K.-H. Kandler, B. Mojsisch, and F.-B. Stammkötter (ed.), *Deitrich von Freiberg: Neue Perspektiven seiner Philosophie, Theologie und Naturwissenschaft*,

Amsterdam and Philadelphia: Grüner, 1999, pp. 69–88 (p. 85); and D. Hedley, *The Iconic Imagination*, New York and London: Bloomsbury, 2016, pp. 47–48.

71 Plotinus, *Enneads*, I.6.9, in Plotinus, *Porphyry on Plotinus; Ennead I*, tr. A.H. Armstrong, Cambridge, MA, and London: Harvard University Press, 1966, p. 261.

72 Klages, *Der Geist als Widersacher der Seele*, pp. 1134–35.

73 Goethe, *Entwurf einer Farbenlehre*, 'Einleitung', in *Werke* [Hamburger Ausgabe], ed. E. Trunz, 14 vols, Hamburg: Wegner, 1948–1960; Munich: Beck, 1981, vol. 13, pp. 324; Goethe, *Theory of Colours*, tr. Charles Lock Eastlake [1840], Cambridge, MA, and London: MIT Press, 1970, p. liii.

74 Müller, *Das verzwistete Ich*, p. 62; cf. Klages, *Der Geist als Widersacher der Seele*, pp. 1133 and 1134, citing Homer, *Odyssey*, book 17, l. 218: 'So the god always brings a like to his own like' (Homer, *The Odyssey*, tr. A. Cook, 2nd edn, New York and London: Norton, 1993, p. 189); and Empedocles, fragment DK31 B109: 'For by earth we see earth, by water water, / by ether bright ether, and by fire flaming fire, / love by love and strife by mournful strife' (J. Barnes (ed.), *Early Greek Philosophy*, Harmondsworth: Penguin, 1987, p. 189).

75 Klages, *Der Geist als Widersacher der Seele*, p. 1133.

76 F. Patrizzi, *Panarchia*, 14: 'De intellectu' (*Nova de universis philosophia*, Ferrara, 1591), fol. 31; cited in E. Cassirer, *The Individual and the Cosmos in Renaissance Philosophy*, tr. M. Domandi, New York, and Evanston, IL: Harper & Row, 1963, pp. 134 and 169.

77 Cited in Cassirer, *The Individual and the Cosmos in Renaissance Philosophy*, p. 169.

78 Klages, *Der Geist als Widersacher der Seele*, p. 1135.

79 M. Weber, *The Protestant Ethic and the Spirit of Capitalism*, tr. T. Parsons, New York; London: Scribner; Allen & Unwin, 1930, p. 232, note 66.

80 For further discussion, see B. Ross, 'The eternal return: Time and time-lessness in P. D. Ouspensky's *Strange Life of Ivan Osokin* and Mircea Eliade's "The secret of Dr. Honigberger"', *Analecta Husserliana: The Yearbook of Phenomenological Research*, vol. 99, *The Cosmos and the Creative Imagination*, ed. A.-T. Tymieniecka and P. Trutty-Coohill, Cham: Springer, 2016, pp. 253–62.

81 A. Peake, *The Labyrinth of Time: The Illusion of Past, Present and Future*, London: Arcturus, 2012.

82 P. S. Loeb, *The Death of Nietzsche's Zarathustra*, Cambridge: Cambridge University Press, 2010.

83 H. Marcuse, *Eros and Civilization: A Philosophical Inquiry into Freud*, London: Routledge & Kegan Paul, 1956, pp. 106–26.

84 Nietzsche, *Thus Spoke Zarathustra*, Part Three, 'The convalescent', §2; *Zarathustra*, tr. Hollingdale, p. 234.

85 Marcuse, *Eros and Civilization*, p. 122.

86 Benjamin, 'Central Park', tr. L. Spencer and M. Harrington, *New German Critique*, Winter 1985, vol. 34, 32–58 (p. 50).

87 C.G. Jung, *The Red Book: Liber Novus*, ed. S. Shamdasani, tr. M. Kyburz, J. Peck, and S. Shamdasani, New York and London: Norton, 2009, p. 244.

88 C.G. Jung, *Symbols of Transformation* [*Collected Works*, vol. 5], tr. R.F.C. Hull, 2nd edn, Princeton, NJ: Princeton University Press, 1967, §253.

89 Jung, *The Red Book*, p. 244.

Chapter 8

Holism and chance

Markets and meaning under neoliberalism

Joshua Ramey

In 2016 I published *Politics of Divination: Neoliberal Endgame and the Religion of Contingency*.[1] The book is an invitation to challenge neoliberal claims for the superiority of markets as a mode of dealing with chance, and to suggest that there have always been and can be again less deadly and more creative ways to engage with the uncertainty in social life than through the medium of markets. My thesis is that a deeper understanding of the social and political stakes of *divination practices* can help to unmask the authoritarian pretensions of neoliberalism in this regard, and open up different ways of reconsidering the political and economic stakes of the role of *chance* in social life. What I mean by divination is, generically, any tradition-bound and systematic practice by which human beings solicit more-than-human knowledge, generally on the basis of chance.[2] I will say more about divination in a moment, but for the moment I need to explain how I understand neoliberalism, in order to set up exactly why I think neoliberalism trades on our understanding of divination in order to persuade us to accept markets as the ultimate form of social order.

Unlike the neoclassical, the neoliberal views markets as information processors. My hypothesis is that the neoliberal experiment in imposing markets and market-like processes on more and more modalities of human cooperation, human need, and human desire has been successful in presenting itself as the only genuine option for social order because markets have a deep resemblance to traditional divination tools. In other words, I argue that neoliberalism has succeeded in presenting itself as common sense partly because it is an ideology that is covertly and unconsciously rooted in ancient ideas about the necessity of divination practices for social order. By divination practices

I mean any tradition-bound and systematic practice by which human beings solicit more-than-human knowledge, generally on the basis of chance — the spill of the entrails, the roll of the bones, the spread of the cards, the flight of birds, the upsurge of intuition by diviners in states of trance.

The fury and frenzy, the effervescence and ferment of markets, and the special form of collective information this chaos is supposed to generate, can be envisioned as a giant surface of divination upon which thousands upon thousands of micro- and macroscopic chances are taken as prices are asked, taken, and asked again. The book contends that our devotion to markets, at least in this particular, 'neoliberal' phase of capitalism, can be characterized as a 'religion of contingency', a ritual practice of determining who can be sacrificed, who is expendable, what must be preserved, and what is to be glorified, on the basis not of the invisible but the *visible* hand of the market, which is chance itself, appearing in the guise of unregulated competition. Whether destructive or creative, peaceful or warlike, every chance is a chance for someone, somewhere, to profit: there are even futures markets in terrorist attacks and natural disasters. When we manage to deplete the earth's carrying capacity for this game, we may all be dead, but someone, somewhere, will be very, very rich.

I'm offering this deliberately hyperbolic picture partly to be provocative, but partly because there is a truth in the hyperbole, a truth about our current hegemonic ideology that is easy to miss because it has largely become common sense. The truth of our complete faith in markets is not a truth that most economists would adhere to — I've never actually met an economist who admits to being a neoliberal, and I doubt whether any of my colleagues in the economics department where I work would dream that markets should completely displace deliberative democracy as a mode of social order. But neoliberalism's influence on public policy and on the most influential economists of the last 30 years is well documented.[3] From its inception in the Mont Pelerin society, a profoundly philosophical movement has seized upon the affordances of markets for deeply sinister ends, a political theory that does not see markets in the instrumental way that most economists tend to, but as ontological ciphers of how reality is, in itself, and how human societies must become in order to conform to that reality.

Neoliberalism glorifies the role of markets as generators of more-than-human knowledge, as what Philip Mirowski calls 'meta-information' processors.[4]

I follow Mirowski's argument that over the last 30 years neoclassical and mainstream orthodox economics has become more neoliberal in this sense. Although variations on this view are everywhere among neoliberals, its clearest formulation must be attributed to the intellectual father of neoliberalism, Friedrich Hayek. In the last period of his career, Hayek was arguing for the point of view that markets don't just process existing economic information but generate new, unforeseeable truths about society (about what is wanted, needed, and possible).[5] Neoliberalism is many things, but I'm mostly interested in this core belief, now taken as common sense, that the imposition of markets or market-like forces in more and more dimensions of human life is a superior form of social coordination, social order, and decision-making than traditional modes of deliberation, debate, consensus formation, or representative democratic processes.

What is 'neo' in neoliberalism, from this point of view, is that whereas classical liberals like Adam Smith thought of markets and market-like processes, and exchange relationships in general, as more or less spontaneous features of human social life (although they were wrong about that — no society has ever been based on barter), neoliberalism sees the state as playing a crucial role in creating and imposing markets and market forces upon society. This is because the essence of the market for them is not that it is a natural way of distributing goods and services, but because it is a cultural ideal of competition that must be engineered and imposed on society from above.[6] From privatization experiments in Chile in the 1970s to the 2008 auctions of the telecommunications bandwidth, from school vouchers to the enforced participation in the health care markets under Obamacare, the neoliberal agenda has been to insinuate markets everywhere, fostering economic competition as a substitute for deliberative democratic processes.

We might debate the merits of any of these experiments. But as long as the underlying ideological presuppositions of neoliberalism are not interrogated, the words of Margaret Thatcher that 'there is no alternative' for genuine social order other than markets and yet more markets will continue to dominate politics, especially in a world where corporate interests have more say than ever before in planning our collective futures (or what is left of them) in a rapidly destabilizing social and natural ecology.

The task of my book is to contribute to undermining neoliberal philosophical presuppositions. Neoliberal capitalism is driven by deeply philosophical commitments that are nevertheless passed off as simple common sense. At the heart of this commitment is a paradox: freedom is found within the constraints of the market. Only market constraints, market discipline, produce genuinely free outcomes. Submission to the laws of the market is the true source of liberty.[7] The problem is not that this view is paradoxical. Most of the enduring philosophical views of human freedom are paradoxical. For Augustine, freedom was submission to God's will; for Spinoza, submission to reason; for Kant, submission to the moral law; for Habermas, submission to the norms of communicative discourse. The problem is the particular neoliberal paradox, which assumes that markets have an *ontological*, indeed *cosmic*, power to embody the truth about human meaning, desire, and purpose.

How is the salience of the particular neoliberal view of freedom justified? The lynchpin of the argument is found in Hayek's work, where he (and Milton Friedman) are quite clear that the problem with so-called 'socialism' — any attempt by the state to pro-actively plan for the economic future — is that it is not responsive enough to unforeseeable contingencies, to the dynamic mutations in supply and demand, cultural and natural changes, rises and falls of favor and disfavor, that mark social life. Their argument, then, is that markets are the only appropriate and only true mediators of chance to human life. That is, markets are the appropriate means by which human expectations encounter the inherent randomness of the universe and in terms of which those expectations must be defined, challenged, and revised. The inherent novelty and differentiation endemic to an indeterminate universe of forces, according to Hayek, is properly mediated to human life only in the form of markets. And if markets, properly constructed, continue to reinforce or exacerbate existing relations of unequal wealth, power, and status, this is simply because markets reflect an evolutionary dynamic that selects those worthy of survival from those unfit for the cosmic future.[8] Markets are in this sense second nature, the economic completion of the work of random selection and adaptive mutation initiated by life itself.

Divinatory markets

Markets, then, are seen as an interaction with chance that results in destiny, a reading of our fates in the vicissitude of market forces. Markets are, that is, tools of divination: a systematic, tradition-bound process used by a community for ascertaining more-than-human knowledge. In the book I examine a range of divination practices, both ancient and contemporary, Western and global, to explore the deep resonance between the role of contemporary markets in neoliberal capitalism and the traditional role of divination rites in social life more generally. I include in my ambit the collective, ritual-trance practices studied by Victor Turner among the Ndembu and by E. E. Evans-Pritchard among the Azande. I studied many other practices, including the ancient auspices of the Daoist and Confucian *I Ching* or book of changes, the global practice of scapulimancy — shoulderbone divination — and a variety of other practices including Yoruban *Ifà*, Tarot reading, dowsing, and the famous Roman practices of divination by observation of the flight paths of birds.

These practices involve the posing of an urgent question — should I go to war? Has someone practiced sorcery? Is now the time to start a new business? — in situations understood to be so enormously complex that they may as well be understood to be redolent with gods, or at least with forces or intentionalities that are radically different to and not in direct communication with human minds. Contemporary market interactions, where buyers and sellers contest the prices of commodities, form a dispersed, collective, continuously iterated practice of inquiry into the unknown, a consultation with the oracle that we, as a market society, collectively constitute. And although it is ultimately an authoritarian sham, the market not only seems to be a divinatory practice but furthermore occupies the place of prestige in social life that divination practices have always held. Like traditional modes of divination, we use markets to continuously contest the results of the oracle, trying again and again for a satisfying answer, for something we can live with (or without). And just as markets can be cornered, rigged, and monopolized, traditional divination rites can also be co-opted by charlatans, rigged by unscrupulous and greedy opportunists, or marred by incorrect procedure. Social mechanisms exist to contest and revise and recast the divinatory event. And yet despite the potential for authoritarian capture, the anthropological record shows that divination techniques are deeply democratic, so much so that they form the basis for almost all contemporary forms of gambling, from dice to roulette to card games. These games are democratic, that is, because they can be played by anyone, and in relation to chance no one has a privileged point of view.

There is an important episode in the history of empire that can clue us into the problem here.[9] The interpretation of lightning and thunder (ceraunomancy) was a divinatory practice commonly used by the college of augurs in Roman society; the college of augurs being the very experts whom the Roman polity relied on in matters of war, politics, and commerce. Rome's struggles with democracy, where the question of what grounds the *authority* of sovereign governance was of profound importance, were deeply embedded in questions surrounding the access to rites of divination. (As observed by many scholars and practitioners, although often practiced by experts, divination is nothing if not contestable — nothing if not a taking and reading of signs open to recasting, replay, revision, and intensely deliberative reflection among all concerned.)

It is this very contention between the *plebs* and *patricians* that led to the secession of the *plebs* to Mons Sacer, a general strike that shut down Rome until certain demands were met. The 'secession of the *plebs*' was not just an exodus from the city of Rome, but also a cleverly targeted occupation: Mons Sacer was the sacred mountain on which the augurs would perform the ritual taking of the auspices. If the *patricians* were to attempt to ignore the *plebs*, and perhaps try to wait it out, eventually the aristocracy of Rome would have to decide what the gods thought about all of this, and thus would be met by the irreverent *plebs*. The demand of the *plebs* for a more democratic society came in the form of access to the rights of divination, since they saw that all civil rights, public and private, were dependent on them. The seat of patrician power was in their exclusive access to the college of augurs and the 'taking of the auspices' performed by the magistrates. For this reason they alone were able to interpret divinatory practices despite the fact that the costs of warfare or failed economic speculation would always be borne by the masses.

The *plebs* mocked the aristocratic reliance upon divinatory authority, and, by doing so, demystified the sacred practice of augury as leaving up to chance grave decisions that would affect entire communities. The *plebs'* demand for inclusion in the taking of the auspices cleverly unmasked the authoritarian capture of chance by the *patricians*. If it was the case that, as the *plebs* had taunted the *patricians*, what was used as the grounds of divine authority were merely random events of chickens feeding, lightning striking, or a particular number of birds in the sky, then the *patricians* ought to be mocked because their authority is derived from either a malicious chicane or a ridiculous human conceit, therefore the *patricians* did not have any authority worth recognizing. But, if the auspices which decided public office, warfare, and law (specifically the laws concerning the payment of debts) *were* in fact divine, then the honor and glory granted by them should include all those they affect. What was at stake for the *plebs* was not just access to divinatory rites and the honors granted by them, but to have a say in what is sacred — to join in the process of providential thinking — in order to have a say in what the future may look like and what sacrifices are worth making. Divination's communal character, insofar as it exists at all, would be not basic or primitive but rather a function of contestation and struggle over the true nature of authority, *over who can be authorized to speak for everyone.*

There are remarkable similarities between the secession of the *plebs* and the OWS movement that ought not to be overlooked. Occupy Wall Street originally intended to occupy the trading room floor at the New York Stock Exchange, the place where the auspices of the global financial system were taken by futures trading — a kind of derivatives trading that determines the value of commodities in the future by way of contracts between exclusive parties, namely those who have the capital to risk — and the demands of OWS were not specific but general. Why was it the case that billions of the aptly named 99% were to suffer the burdens of a financial market which decided the future of humanity and its environmental conditions without the 99% having a voice in these decisions at all?

Gaming chance

There is something deeply democratic about chance, and that is part of why market-based society seems to have so much popular appeal, at least in the United States. Anyone can get lucky, anyone can get a break. Jackson Lear, in his monumental study *Something for Nothing: Luck in America*, contends that gambling maintains such an important place in American culture because of the association of chance with *grace*, with a free gift of potential change in status that is available to anyone, regardless of pre-existing arrangements of wealth and power, regardless of how much of a winner or loser you've been up to that point.[10] And as David Graeber and many others have shown, divination in the form of the casting of lots also has an extraordinary relation to the history of democratic experimentation, from the lots cast to determine the Athenian assembly to the law, still on the books in the state of Arizona, that in runoffs between candidates for certain governmental positions, a tie is decided by the draw of the higher card from a deck.[11]

My argument is that neoliberalism draws heavily upon our cultural and historical familiarity with divination, and with the importance of divination for both religious and democratic aspirations, in order to justify its celebrations of markets. If it is in markets that we truly find our chances, find grace, and discover the lineaments of true democracy — where no one is chosen or not by nature, where all have a chance — then even if markets continue to massively fail us and wound us, to what other secular god will we turn? If we believe that markets are the temple of chance, then it is to markets that we must sacrifice, and market outcomes we must praise.

Marketplace games are disastrously, even catastrophically limited games, externalizing the ecological and social costs of profit-seeking in a way that has imperiled life on this planet. But the sacred identity of such games is *more generic* than economic activity can capture, and consciousness of the role of chance in social life must be expanded beyond the purview of the market and beyond the usual dismissal of divination based on its supposed irrationality and mystification. Other stories incorporating chance can be told, other meanings made, other affordances encouraged and fostered. There are other politics of divination than that dominated by the rule of profit. But for progressive politics to advance beyond its rationalistic modernist limitations, and to imagine another politics of divination, will require conceptions of individuality, responsibility, agency, choice, and meaning that more fully acknowledge the interdependency, uncertainty, fragility, and contingency of our plans in the face of chance. Only then can other relations to chance be cultivated than those currently embodied by market-based divinations of value through price alone.

To understand this we need a brief discussion of the role of games in social life. In his brilliant 1958 study, *Man, Play, and Games*, Roger Caillois proposed that games and play constitute an important force in the establishment and maintenance of social life:

> Games discipline instincts and institutionalize them. For the time that they afford formal and limited satisfaction, they educate, enrich, and immunize the mind against their virulence. At the same time, they are made fit to contribute usefully to the enrichment of the establishment of various patterns of culture.[12]

Games are meant to be a supplement to, and not a substitute for, social life in general. Yet the point of understanding games and play, for Caillois, is that social life in general attempts to imitate or bring into being the principles aspired to by ideal games. The ideal game for a modern, democratic polity would be one that perfectly subordinates the role of chance to that of merit, the role of unforeseeable contingency to the rule of maximum reward for maximum displays of excellence. 'That is why political reformers ceaselessly try to devise more equitable types of competition and hasten their implementation', Caillois puts it.[13]

Caillois proposed that games of chance (of *alea*, in Greek) were one among four types that could define the range of games played by human societies. The other three include games of make-believe or imitation (*mimicry*), games of competitive skill (*agôn*), and games of vertigo (*ilinx*, the Greek term for whirlpool). Historically, Caillois notes that democratic societies have tended to emphasize games of *agôn* and *alea* over those of *mimicry* and *ilinx*. Societies (typically pre-modern) that search for a sense of justice and order through identification with transcendent powers — gods, ancestral spirits, or animal totems — tend to use rituals of imitation (including masks) and the inducement of vertigo (*ilinx*) through dance and consciousness-altering substances, to allow more-than-human powers to become felt as present to, and authoritative for, the life of the community. One way or another, games allow hierarchies to be justified and order maintained in a context of mutual recognition that the sources of life, health, and continuity transcend and include the entire community. As the outcome of games, the lot of each becomes something that can be meaningfully accepted. Unlike traditional societies, those with egalitarian aspirations attempt to establish a just social order partly by allowing for the establishment of rank through agonistic games of competition establishing merit or worthiness, and partly through games of chance which acknowledge that the ability to compete is itself a matter of contingent placements of birth, innate talent and intelligence, family support, and other ways in which individuals are differentiated by unaccountable forces that precede and produce their stations in life.

In a democratic society, as Caillois puts it, the role of competitive games of skill and those of chance are understood to be 'contradictory yet complementary'.[14] That is to say, there is never a stable synthesis, let alone a perfect identity between fair chances and equal merit. And this synthesis is largely a failed project. Although modernity tries to 'enlarge the domain of regulated competition, or merit, at the expense of birth and inheritance, or chance', this project remains unfulfilled — 'remote and improbable', for Caillois, because it is an 'evolution which is reasonable, just and favorable [only] to the *most capable*' (emphasis added).[15] Those unable to compete are tempted to rebel against modernity's offer of inclusion through merit, and are led deeper and deeper into superstitious relations to chance. As Caillois puts it:

> As for the avarice today observed in the pursuit of good fortune, it probably compensates for the continuous tension involved in modern competition. Whoever despairs of his own resources is led to trust in destiny. Excessively rigorous competition discourages the timid and tempts them to rely on external powers. By studying and utilizing heavenly powers over chance, they try to get the reward they doubt can be won by their own qualities, by hard work and steady application.[16]

To overcome the superstition that thinks it can read chance as destiny, societies with egalitarian aspirations are caught in the following difficulty. True distributive justice, giving to each what each is due, must always in some sense be unequal if there are unequal chances for the development of merit and the proving of worth (to say nothing of the fact long noticed by communist social theory that different individuals may have very different needs and requirements in order to contribute). And if chance is objective, not an illusion but a feature of reality, then the so-called playing field between competitors can never, in principle, be perfectly leveled. Agonistic competition for the establishment of value and worth can never completely eliminate the chance differences between the advantages of opponents. But neither can chance ever fully obscure the sense that some individuals are inherently more worthy of honor than others.

As long as the overcoming of the chances of birth and placement by effort and merit eludes us, either in games or in social life generally, the unstable tension between the roles of chance and achievement threatens to undo the fabric of egalitarian societies. And Caillois argued that under social conditions where fair competition is perceived as being too difficult, games of chance take on inordinate importance and become perverse, leading to superstition, a reliance on 'external powers' of chance and destiny for success. Caillois writes:

> [*Alea*] leaves hope in the dispossessed that free competition is still possible in the lowly stations in life… That is why, to the degree that *alea* of birth loses its traditional supremacy and regulated competition becomes dominant, one sees a parallel development and proliferation of a thousand secondary mechanisms designed to bring sudden success out of turn to the rare winner.[17]

Caillois's argument in *Man, Games, and Play* was that the role of competition must not be excessive or unfair, lest modern societies devolve into barbaric inequality and provoke revolt. But dreams of a mid-twentieth-century Keynesian, democratic-socialist compromise with capitalism eventually lost to the neoliberal argument that markets could manage themselves and thus manage democratic aspirations automatically. A dogma that 'free markets' would adjudicate all claims to worthiness (value) directly on the basis of impersonal market forces (unforeseeable contingent variability of supply and demand) became the neoliberal superstition of our times. It is as if the neoliberal era, with its championing of markets as a substitute for social policy, and market tests as a proof of merit, claimed markets could identify games of *alea* directly with those of *agôn*, and that markets had the power to honor both competitive merit and unmerited luck, in the same fell swoop.

I argue that this identification of markets with *both* the discernment of genuine merit *and* the honoring of chance is possible only on the basis of an equivocation in the neoliberal era between markets and traditional forms of divination. This is the sense of my thesis that markets are not really, but *really seem* to be, divinatory and thus divine. In economic life, which is supposed to be the place, according to champions of the market, where *agôn* and *alea* finally stabilize and synthesize, the primary engines through which marketplace activity occurs are the games most excluded from social valorization: mimicry and *ilinx*. The giving and taking of prices — especially in the speed and intensity of complex finance — is a complex game of *imitation* in which one tries to demand the price that one thinks the average person would accept in a given moment (thus the key role of imitation), and the ability to propose the right price is a matter of surrendering oneself to the vertiginous whorl that is the market itself (*ilinx*). In this way, markets present themselves as the necessary supplement to other egalitarian processes such as elections. But this is done through those affects — ecstatic imitation and sympathetic intuition — through which humans attempt to surpass the need for deliberation and contestation upon which democratic processes depend. This is especially clear in the intensity of the trading pit, where buyers and sellers must use their 'animal spirits' to persuade one another to give and take prices beyond what is probable or reasonable to expect. (As trader and philosopher Elie Ayache explains, each time a price is agreed to, the entire market is re-created, since given the saturation of information, there would be no trading at all if the market could not be re-created each time, beyond probability, beyond the reasonable expectations held by all traders in common.)[18]

The 'state' in which one divines is precisely a state of mimicry and ilinx, since the skilled diviner must enter into a state of openness to potential meaning that is accessible only through the alteration of consciousness, the expansion of consciousness, through both sympathetic and symbiotic relations to the clients seeking wisdom and to the spirits embodied in the oracular techniques and traditions with which the diviner works. In this way, our current dependence upon markets as a form of social order reveals a very deep impasse in modernity, one Caillois identified as the rejection or repression of the role of games of mimicry and *ilinx* as valid, justifiable modes of human activity. In some sense the reason that *agôn-alea* remains an unstable pairing, in modernity, is that the roles of mimicry and *ilinx* are rejected as irrational and without legitimate social purpose. The tension between the slow, sober processes of rational deliberation and the ecstatic, impassioned cunning of marketplace activity threatens to tear egalitarian society apart. But this is a problem much older than capitalist culture, and cultures that integrate divination practices into what it means to deliberate may help us to understand ourselves — and to act — better than we do.

Divining otherwise

To evoke divination practices as a framing of complex contemporary problems may seem spooky or outré, especially when we now use big data and complex algorithms to place bets on possible futures that seem grounded in empirically verified probabilities. But the probable does not exhaust the possible, and in fact profitability (especially on the massively capitalized derivatives market) depends crucially on our models of future states *not* being ever completely accurate. Bear traders, for example, can only short the market if the consensus view of probability is wrong.[19] And it is precisely the glut of information provided by big data which diminishes the possibility of what is called information arbitrage, making large gains in financial speculation extremely difficult. (The primary arguments used to justify the massive amounts of capital that are locked up in the derivatives market is not that it creates new wealth, but that shifting bets on options and futures *reveals important information* about where the economy is and where it is going, making the derivatives market in particular an especially important, perhaps the key, pseudo-divinatory practice.)[20]

The problem, of course, is that the pressure that is placed on firms and nations by hedge funds to show profitability, to show efficiencies, and so on, derives from the interests of the largest bondholders or holders of options. That interest is profitability, which may or may not reflect the interest of the general public, the nation state, global peace, or the ecosystems upon which industry and finance survive. And it is precisely here that we desperately need a post-capitalist future in which power does not devolve exclusively to the largest firms and the command over labor and capital that their holdings represent.

By figuring contemporary neoliberal commitments to markets as a subspecies of a general human commitment to divination practices, I argue that while neoliberalism may be right that *some* collective practice of divination is necessary, it is not necessary that this practice be figured in and as markets. While marketplace divinations are geared exclusively toward the discernment of what is profitable in the nearest term possible, more expansive and capacious forms of divination would enquire as to how clear and present human needs, desires, frustrations, and longings might themselves require modification in view of those human and non-human others to which we are related by interdependency and not by rent-seeking, bartering, or zero-sum competition.

Such non-contractual, non-hierarchical, subtle and often ambiguous relational interdependencies are those that black theory, Marxist, feminist, queer, and deep ecological thinkers have been trying to draw our attention to for many years. They are the interdependencies traditional divination practices seek to render tractable for human communities in relation to the complex and ultimately obscure forces present to us in such constituencies as (in no particular order) the world of other less-able and less-wealthy human beings than those who can compete in the marketplace, as well as animals, plant life, ecological niches, seasonal changes, ancestral spirits, unconscious archetypes, and other potencies of suffering and joy calling for attention below the reaches of the conscious mind.[21]

You and I may disagree about who or what should be on this list worthy of our attention and care and fidelity. But the problem, from my perspective, is not that contemporary neoliberalism denies the reality of non-human persons and powers, or the influence of their unforeseeable relations to our plans and projects. The problem is that neoliberalism is an ideology that believes, with totalitarian and authoritarian certainty, that markets and market processes can dominate, control, and order the unknown once and for all. Neoliberalism has locked up the god of chance and thrown away the key of uncertainty. The ecological, social, and psychological costs of this particular politics of divination and this particular religion of contingency are increasingly clear. The question remains whether we will continue with neoliberalism deeper into the social and ecological death it entails, or whether we will re-animate the archive of traditional practices, in order to return to a place we truly cannot leave: an earth-bound experiment with subtle, nuanced, and open-ended practices of reading chance aloud, together.

Notes

1 *Politics of Divination: Neoliberal Endgame and the Religion of Contingency* (Rowman and Littlefield, Intl., 2016). This paper is a précis of the arguments of the book, and was presented as a talk at the conference, 'Holism: Possibilities and Problems: An International Interdisciplinary Conference,' September 8–10, 2017.
2 Anthony Thorley, Chantal Allison, Petra Stapp, and John Wadsworth, 'Clarifying divinatory dialogue: A proposal for a distinction between practitioner divination and essential divination,' in *Divination: Perspectives for a New Millennium*, edited by Patrick Curry (Farnham, UK: Ashgate Publishing Limited, 2010), 252–253.
3 See especially Philip Mirowski, *Never Let a Serious Crisis Go to Waste: How Neoliberalism Survived the Financial Meltdown* (London: Verso, 2013).
4 Ibid.
5 Friedrich Hayek, *Law, Legislation, and Liberty*, vol. 1 (Chicago: University of Chicago Press, 1973).
6 See especially Michel Foucault, *The Birth of Biopolitics* (New York: Palgrave Macmillan, 2008), chaps. 5–7.
7 See Friedrich Hayek, *The Road to Serfdom* (Chicago: University of Chicago Press, 1944) and Milton Friedman, *Capitalism and Freedom* (Chicago: University of Chicago Press, 1962).
8 Michel Foucault already made clear, in his 1978–79 lectures, that the exacerbation of wealth inequality would be no argument against the value of imposing market forces on all of social life, since already for the German Ordoliberal school — highly influential on Hayek and subsequent neoliberal ideology — inequality helps to facilitate and maintain competition, which is the essence of the social life neoliberalism aims to produce. Foucault, *The Birth of Biopolitics*, chaps. 5–7.

9 I owe the details of the account of the secession of the *plebs* and its impli-cation for my argument to the unpublished research of Adam Cope, and I owe to Adam, as well, the observations about the connections between the secession of the *plebs* and the tactics of Occupy Wall Street.

10 Jackson Lear, *Something for Nothing: Luck in America* (New York: Viking Books, 2003).

11 David Graeber, *The Democracy Project: A History, A Crisis, A Movement* (New York: Spiegel & Grau, 2013).

12 Roger Caillois, *Man, Games, and Play*, translated by Meyer Barash (Urbana: University of Illinois Press, 2001), 55.

13 Ibid., 114.

14 Ibid.

15 Ibid.

16 Ibid., 48.

17 Ibid., 114.

18 Elie Ayache, *The Blank Swan: The End of Probability* (New York: Wiley, 2010).

19 For a clear exposition of this point, following on from Ayache's work, see Arjun Appadurai, *Banking on Words: The Failure of Language in the Age of Derivative Finance* (Chicago: University of Chicago Press, 2015).

20 See Dick Bryan and Michael Rafferty, *Capitalism with Derivatives: A Political Economy of Financial Derivatives, Capital, and Class* (New York: Palgrave Macmillan, 2006).

21 For an analysis of how capitalism and money constrict our ability to attend to or develop awareness of real but unprofitable forces, see Philip Goodchild, *Capitalism and Religion: The Price of Piety* (London: Routledge, 2001).

Index

Note: Figures are denoted by *italic* text and notes by "n" and the number of the note after the page number, e.g., 163n12 refers to note number 12 on page 163. The lengthy list of figures against "geometry, of wholeness" and "wholeness, geometry of" are explained on page ix.

1227: Treatise on nomadology – the war machine 52, 55, 60

À la Recherche du Temps Perdu 28
Absolute, the 31
absolute religion 56
abstract idea of the State 52–59, 63, 65, 69, 71
acategoriality 158–159
achievement 203
actual, the 39, 40, 41, 114, 120, 161, 162n3
affect/affectivity 66, 108, 155, 175, 204; and the edusemiotic self 104, 110, 116, 120, 122; of self on self 122; and symptomatology 85, 90, 91, 93, 97
agôn/agonistic competition 201, 203, 204
alchemy 5, 11, 23, 24, 31, 32; and the edusemiotic self 106–107, 109–110, 111, 112, 119; and exceptional experiences 151, 159–160, 161, 163n12
alea 201, 202, 203, 204
alliances, between different fields 67–68
alternative spiritualities, therapies, and work practices 1
analytical psychology 11, 52, 67, 68, 75n26, 185; and symptomatology 91, 97, 98
anamnesis 31

Anaxagoras 180–181, 182, 190n67
anima mundi 109, 139
anomalous experience 26, 27
Answer to Job 35, 37
Anthropocene, the 9
Anti-Oedipus 4, 28–29
anti-Semitism 21
apocatastasis 31, 37
applied psychoanalysis 82
archetypal aspect of existence 88
archetypal experiences 114–115
archetypal imagery 36, 89, 90, 91, 119, 120, 122
archetypal phenomena 132
archetypal shadow 122
archetypes 32, 33, 114, 119, 120, 158, 206; and anima 69; of collective unconscious 24–25, 103, 104, 110, 113; Jungian 85, 90, 91, 105, 106, 145, 149–150; as ruling powers 115; as structural elements of psyche 105; and synchronicities 153–154; of transformation 119; and unus mundus 150–151; virtual 12; of wholeness 31, 89, 103, 104
art, modern 52, 67, 68, 69, 74n16
aspect monism 162n3; *see also* dual-aspect monism; neutral monism
Asprem, Egil 26, 35, 36

assemblages 85, 104, 107
authoritarianism 193, 197, 198, 199, 206–207
autonomous unconscious 91, 98

background reality 150
baseline correlations 156
becoming 75n22, 89, 97, 170, 172; and Being 173; and the edusemiotic self 112, 114–115, 117, 118, 122; and holism 27, 29, 37, 39, 41; of Jung's characters 85, 90; process of 116–117; *see also* rhizome
becoming estranged 64–66
becoming-active 173
becoming-imperceptible 71
becoming-majoritarian 59
becoming-minoritarian 59
becoming-other 12, 116, 122
becoming-reactive 173
becoming-revolutionary 59
becoming-self 102–107, 110, 116, 122
becoming-woman 110
Benjamin, Walter 184
Bergson, Henri 6, 27, 112
Bergsonism 4
bidirectionality 149, 154
bifurcation 133–135, *135*, *136*, 139, 140
binary opposites 109, 118; *see also* dualisms/duality
Birth of Tragedy, The 181
body without organs 4
Bohm, David 122, 144, 162n3
bounded system 1
bounded whole 65

Caillois, Roger 201–202, 203–204, 205
capitalism 194, 196, 197, 203–204
capture 55–56, 58, 62, 64; authoritarian 198, 199
causal closure, of the physical 142, 143
Central Park 184
centralization 30
centrifugal power 173
chance 13, 14, 152, 158, 193–208
chaos/chaotic states 12, 67, *138*, 194
chess 57, 58
classical theism 10, 34, 35, 45n5

clinical domain 102, 117; and symptomatology 80, 81, 82, 84, 85, 94, 98
clinicians of civilization 83
closed wholes 28
cobweb plot 133, 134, *137*, 140
Codex Fejérváry-Mayer 126, *129*, 131, 140
coincidence phenomena 86, 109, *156*, 156–157, 158, 160
Coldness and cruelty 80
collective assemblages 104
collective culture 86
collective information 194
collective level, of experience 62, 88, 94, 115
collective opinion 62, 63–64
collective projection 61–62
collective unconscious 11, 24, 68, *145*, 150; and edusemiotic self 103, 110–111, 113, 114, 121–122; and symptomatology 85, 90, 92, 93, 98
common man 61
communication, transversal 109
competition 194, 195, 201, 202, 203–204, 206, 207n8
complementarity 107–108, 148–149
completeness, of the physical 142, 143
complexes 85, 103
complexity theory 1–2, 9
compositional dual-aspect monism 144
conceptual personae 62
conceptual world 60, 62, 69
conjunctions 23, 31
connectedness 147, 161
conscious ego 24–25, 106, 160
consciousness: cultural 118; ego- 43; empirical 37; minoritarian 59; subjective 149–150
consciousness research 12
consequent nature, of the divine 40
constructivism 10, 110
contingency 13, 194, 201, 207
Convalescent, The 169, 170, 171, 183
correlations 127, 143, 144, 146, 149, 151–155, 156–157, 157–158
correspondence 38, 82, 119, 130, 140, 150, 153

cosmic mandalas 140; *see also* Codex
    Fejérváry-Mayer; Kalachakra
    mandala
cosmography 126–127
cosmology 24, 31–32, 34, 35, 126–127,
    131–132
cosmos 168, 169, 174, 180
counter-actualisation 114
countercultural movements 1
creativity 7, 9, 10, 72, 87, 139, 180; and
    edusemiotic self 102–103, 112, 117,
    120–121; and holism 27, 29, 32, 37,
    38, 39, 40
creed 56, 61, 73n11; of Deleuze's
    ethics 117
critical, the 80–81, 90, 94, 98
critical holism 7, 8
culture 1, 2, 5, 6, 9, 63; and edusemiotic
    self 115–116, 118, 121; and markets
    200, 201, 205; and symptomatology
    86, 92, 93–94

decompositional dual-aspect monism 12
deficit correlations 154, 157
Deleuze and the Unconscious 5–6, 14n1
deliberative democracy 194
depersonalization 116
depth psychology 43, 51, 104, 105
derivatives market 205
desire 6, 87, 109–110, 193, 196, 206
desiring-production 105–106
determinism 29, 152
deterritorialization 94
diagnosis 80, 102, 117
dictator States 54
difference 10, 13, 28, 86, 87, 172;
    and edusemiotic self 107, 108,
    112, 113
Difference and Repetition 6, 11, 171, 172;
    and 'image of thought' and State-form
    52, 62, 63, 65, 75n25
differentiation 12, 38, 71, 75n25, 196
diremption, of modern man 61
disembodiment 64, 65, 75n21, 175;
    see also embodiment
disenchantment 7, 13, 74n19, 75n21; and
    eternal recurrence 167–168, 174, 184;
    and holism 20, 26, 27, 33, 34, 36, 42;

and holistic enchantment 167–168,
    174, 184
dispersal 139
dissimilarity 13, 171
dissociation phenomena *156*, 157
dissolution 65, 90, 109
distributive justice 203
divination 13, 14, 122, 193–194,
    197–199, 200–201, 204–207
divine, the 7, 110, 116, 144; and holism
    34–35, 39, 40, 42, 45n5
domination 54, 59
dramatisation 12, 93, 120
dreams 103, 110, 119, 127, *131*, 138,
    158; and symptomatology 85, 94,
    95–96, 96–97
dual-aspect monism 12, 143–145,
    146, 154
dual-aspect thinking 143, 161–162n1
dualisms/duality 2, 3, 39, 139, 140, 181;
    and edusemiotic self 112, 118, 121;
    and exceptional experiences 143, 151,
    155; *see also* binary opposites
Dühring, Eugen 168–169
dying man 88–89

Eastern thought 9
ecology 2, 7, 20, 21, 132; and markets
    196, 200, 206, 207
economics 195, 204
ecosystems 1, 206
education 6, 7, 8, 11, 102; psychological
    67, 69, 71; self- 103–104, 120
edusemiotic self 102–122, *108*, *121*
EE (exceptional experiences) 9, 12–13,
    142–163, *145*, *156*
ego, conscious 24–25, 106, 160
ego-consciousness 43
elementary similarity 13, 177–178,
    179–180
embodiment 54–55, 69, 114, 121, 122,
    201, 205; *see also* disembodiment
empiricism 25, 26, 29, 30, 37, 38, 68, 113
enchanted Others 33
enchantment 13, 74n19; holistic 167–192
encounter, the 52, 66
energy 37, 42, 105–106
entelechy 31

environmentalism 9
epistemic levels of reality 144–145
epistemology 1, 2, 3, 8, 70–71, 148–149, 151, 155
Eros 109–110
Eros and Civilization: A Philosophical Inquiry into Freud 183
esotericism 5, 9, 36, 44
Essays Critical and Clinical 11, 81
esse in anima 7, 33
essences 91, 111–112, 176, 177, 178; and holism 28, 29, 37
essentialism 21, 30
estrangement 9, 52, 64–66, 67, 70, 72
eternal recurrence/eternal return 5, 13, 168, 169–172, 172–173, 173–174, 176, 183, 184
ethical ambivalence, of holism 20–45
ethical responsibility 116
Ethics (book) 172, 187n24
ethics (concept) 11–12, 58, 65; of integration 115–119
etiology 82
exceptional experiences (EE) 9, 12–13, 142–163, *145*, *156*
excess correlations 154, 156–157
excess libido 92
exchange relationships 195
excluded third 105, 107
exclusion 4, 7, 53, 60, 64, 68
experience: acategorial 158–159; anomalous 26, 27; archetypal 114–115; collective level of 62, 88, 94, 115; empirical 25, 38; exceptional 9, 12–13, 142–163, *145*, *156*; immanent 9, 12, 13, 159; multiplicities of 8, 14n1; mystical 104–105, 158; numinous 26, 27, 35; reified 13, 157, 158, 160; relational 13, 157, 158, 160; synchronistic 33, 112, 157–158
experiential learning 11
experiential wholes 29
experimentation 38, 86, 87, 98, 110, 113, 118, 200
exteriority 7, 52, 57–58, 69, 70, 120
external phenomena *156*, 156, 157
external power 201–202, 203
external relations 30, 41

extramundane, the 25–26, 52, 56, 64, 66, 67–71
extreme contingency 13, 14, 152, 158, 193–208
eyes of the mind 110–111

finalism 29
financial markets 13, 14, 193–208
form of exteriority 52, 69, 70, 76n31
fractal geometry 12, 130–131, 132, 133, 139
freedom, human 186n16, 196
future wholes 10, 29, 30–31, 32, 36, 37, 41, 42
futures trading 199

games/gaming chance 200–205
Geist 2, 23, 81, 106, 109, 119, 158, 160; and eternal recurrence 168, 174, 175, 179, 180, 182
gender 9
geometry: fractal 12, 130–131, 132, 133, 139; of wholeness 125–140, *126*, *127*, *128*, *129*, *130*, *131*, *134*, *135*, *136*, *137*, *138*
German holism 21
gnosis 5, 11–12, 109, 110, 114, 120
Gnosticism 5, 39, 110, 121, 139
Go 57
Goethe, Johann Wolfgang von 167–168
Guattari, Félix 4, 5, 10, 28–29, 51, 73n10

habits of thought 60
Handwriting and Character 178
Hayek, Friedrich 13, 195, 196
hearing 11, 90, 91, 98
Hegel, Georg Wilhelm Friedrich 31, 44–45n4, 183
Heidegger, Martin 13, 170–171, 174, 175, 180, 188n40
hermeneutics 81, 132
Hermeticism 7, 27, 31, 37–38, 103, 109, 160
hidden world 91–92
historicism 21
holism: and chance 193–208; critical 7, 8; ethical ambivalence of 20–45;

German 21; organicistic 7, 30–32; rhizomatic/transversal 7
Holism: Possibilities and Problems 7–8
holistic enchantment, and eternal recurrence 167–192
holistic reality *145*, 147
holistic thought 2–3, 7, 9, 20, 21–30, 36, 42
homoiomeries 18, 182
homoiōsis/homology 180, 181–182, 189n59
human freedom 186n16, 196
human wholeness 22–23

I Ching 119, 127, *130*, 197
Idea 176
ideal games 201
idealised State 61
idealism, Platonic 176
identity 4, 13, 87, 113, 200, 202; and eternal recurrence 171–172, 175, 179; and external experiences 153–154, 158; and holistic enchantment 171–172, 175, 179
ilinx 201, 202
illness 83, 84
image of thought 11, 51, 52, 60–71; *see also* rhizome
images, impression and intuitive 178
imitation, games of 201, 202, 204–205
immanence 10, 106, 109, 110, 157–161, 163n10; and holism 22, 26, 35, 36, 37, 40–41; plane of 4, 34, 38, 76n28, 106, 110, 118, 121; pure 4, 10, 33–34, 38, 40, 44, 109; secret 106
immanent experiences 9, 12, 13, 159
immediate inner experience 64, 68–69
imperceptible, the 91, 104
impersonal transcendental field 109
impression images 178
incarnation, of the transcendental field of the collective unconscious 114
included third 11, 105, 111, 150
individual (Jung) 53, 55, 58, 59, 61, 62, 63, 65, 66
individual development 3
individual psyche 3; *see also* psyche, the
individual wholeness 23, 25, 44n2

individuation 3, 11, 52–53, 104, 110, 160; and archetypes 114–115, 150–151, 158; axiom of Maria Prophetissa as 107; as becoming-self 102–107, 116, 117, 119, 122; and holism 23, 25–26, 43; and symptomatology 76n27, 76n30, 86–87
induced correlations 154–155
information processing 74n18, 193
inner, the 68–69, 70–71, 148
inner psychic integration 23
inner/outer binary 69
integrated mind 23–24, 160
integrated whole 112
integration, ethics of 115–119
intelligence 114, 202
intentionality 65, 152, 163n9
interconnectedness 2, 26
interiority 7, 55–56, 56–57, 57–58, 60, 68, 69, 70
internal phenomena *156*, 156
internal relations 7, 30–32
intuitions 3, 27, 61, 114, 169, 182, 194, 204; and symptomatology 92–93, 95
intuitive images 178
invisible, the 91–92, 104, 106, 108–109, 110–111, 118, 120
irrationality 26, 200; *see also* rationality
irregular, the 58
irrepresentable, the 11, 26, 104

Jenkins, Barbara 6, 9
Jungian archetypes 85, 90, 91, 105, 106, 145, 149–150

Kalachakra mandala 126–127, *128*, 131, 140
Kant, Immanuel 5, 9, 38, 74n20, 114, 158, 160, 196
Kerslake, Christian 5–6, 14n1, 75n25, 80, 163n10
Klages, Ludwig 13, 173–176, 177–180, 182–183
knowledge 5, 11–12, 109, 110, 114, 120; more-than-human 14, 193, 195, 197
Krause, Karl Christian Friedrich 36

language 51, 59, 90, 94–95, 115, 118–119
learning 11, 80, 94; and edusemiotic self
    102, 104, 112, 113, 114, 118
levelling down, statistical 53
libido 92, 105–106, 110, 185
literature 80–81, 83–84, 86
local realism 146–148
Logic of Sense 40
Logos 28, 61, 110, 120, 175

macrocosm 24, 25, 31, 37–38, 177
major literature 95–96
majoritarian 54–55, 59
majority 54, 59, 71, 72n4, 95
make-believe, games of 201, 202,
    204–205
Man, Play, and Games 201
mandala symbolism 126, 127, *130*, *131*
Mandelbrot, Benoit 12, 131–132, 133
Mandelbrot set 133–135, *134*, *135*, *136*,
    137, *138*, 139
Marcuse, Herbert 183
market forces 195, 197, 204, 207n8
marketplace games 200–201
markets, financial 13, 14, 193–208
masochism 75n25, 80
mass man 11, 51–52, 53, 54, 55, 58, 60,
    64, 69–70
mass opinion 62, 63–64
mass projection 61–62
mass-mindedness 53, 54
material vitalism 7
material world 25, 111, 139, 153, 154,
    155, 159
materialism 176
mathematics 104–105, 140
mathesis universalis 118–119, 121
matter 2, 3, 4, 26, 56, 176, 185; and
    edusemiotic self 106, 112; and
    exceptional experiences 145, 146,
    148; and wholeness 139, 140; *see also*
    mind-matter correlations
measurement 146–147, 148, 149,
    154
mental, the 12, 13, 34, 143–161, *145*
mental-physical correlations 143, 144,
    149, 157–158
merit 201, 202–203, 204

metaphysics 7, 26–27, 38, 40, 42, 144,
    170–171
methodology 8, 53, 61, 98, 175
methods 71, 104, 113, 116, 117, 152, 175
microcosm 24, 25, 31, 37–38, 177
microphysics 149
mimicry 201, 204–205
mind, integrated 23–24, 160
mind-matter correlations 143, 144, 149,
    151–155, 157–158
minor literature 11, 80, 94–98
minoritarian consciousness 59
minority politics 11, 97, 98
models of reality 155
modern art 52, 67, 68, 69, 74n16
modern differentiation 38
modernity 44n2, 52, 64, 72n3, 202, 205
monism 12, 143–145, 146, 154, 162n3
Mons Sacer 198
more-than-human knowledge 14, 193,
    195, 197
multiplicities 8, 11, 14n1, 107–115, *108*,
    117, 120, 122
mundus potentialis 118
Mysterium Coniunctionis 23, 32, 151,
    159–161
mystical experiences 104–105, 158
mystical thought 7, 9

nature 2, 7, 12, 30, 34, 140, 167, 187n24;
    and edusemiotic self 102, 104, 105,
    106, 108, 109; and exceptional experi-
    ences 142, 149, 150
nature–culture network 121
Nazism 20–21, 173–174
neoliberal capitalism 194, 196, 197
neoliberalism 13–14, 193–194, 195,
    196–197, 203–204, 206, 207n8
neo-Platonism 39, 114, 158
neutral language 12
neutral monism 143–144
newborn infant 88–89
Nietzsche, Friedrich 5, 13, 61, 70, 82, 87,
    167–192
Nietzsche and Philosophy 171–172
nihilism 14, 173
Nobody 54, 59
nomadicism 59

noncausal correspondence 153
non-identity thinking 180
nonlocal correlations 146
non-personal power 85, 87
non-rational, the 26
noology 70
normal man 59, 73n6
numinous experience 26, 27, 35

objective psyche 103
objective unconscious 149–150
object-recognition 68
occultism 6
Occupy Wall Street (OWS) 199
Of Cosmogonic Eros 174–175
one world *see* unus mundus
one-sided image 52, 61, 72
one-sidedness 25, 66
ontic levels of reality 144–145
open society 118
open systems 33
open whole 4, 8, 32–42
open-ended creativity 37
opposites 105, 106, 109, 118, 174–175,
    182; coincidence of 86, 109, 158, 160;
    union of 22–23, 135, 158
ordinary correlations 156
organicism 4, 7, 10, 73n10; and holism
    29–30, 30–32, 37–38, 41, 42
organisation 10; invisible plane of 106;
    of relations 51, 53, 65, 66, 68, 69; of
    thought 51
organism 1, 4, 51, 61, 65, 75n22, 176;
    and holism 28, 30, 31, 41
original wholes 10, 29, 30–31, 32, 36,
    37, 41, 42
otherness 9, 86
outside thought 70, 71
OWS (Occupy Wall Street) 199

panentheism 7, 10, 32–42, 45n6, 45n7
pantheism 10, 33–35, 45n5, 45n6,
    74n20
parts 4, 65, 86, 106, 144, 168; and holism
    21, 24–25, 28–29, 29–30, 31, 32, 36
pathology 3, 25, 61, 84, 110
patricians 198–199
Pauli, Wolfgang 12, 68, 111, 118, 139

Pauli-Jung conjecture 12, 142–163,
    145, 156
Peirce, Charles S. 102, 107, 111
percept 11, 80, 90–94, 97, 98
perception 13, 34, 104, 114, 122, 155,
    157, 179
peripheral totality 86
personal transformation 5
personality 24, 25, 86–87
phenomenological typology, of
    exceptional experiences 155–157, *156*
philosophical concepts 8, 81, 145–146
photon pair 146
physical, the 12, 13, 34, 142, 143,
    144, 150, 151; and immanence 157,
    158, 160, 161; and mind–matter
    correlations 153, 154; and Pauli-Jung
    conjecture *145*, 146; and synchronicity
    153–154; and transcendence 157, 158,
    160, 161
physical reality/physical world 23, 25,
    111, 139; and exceptional experiences
    146–148, 153, 154, 155, 159
physicalism 142, 143, 158
physics 12, 33, 68, 111; and exceptional
    experiences 142, 144–145, 146,
    148–149, 150, 152, 157, 162n6
physis 139, 140
plane of immanence 4, 34, 38, 76n28,
    106, 110, 118, 121
plane of Nature 106
Platonic idealism 176
Platonism 28, 33, 38, 39, 111, 171
plebs 198–199, 208n9
plurality 86
political economy 9
*Politics of Divination: Neoliberal
    Endgame and the Religion of
    Contingency* 13–14, 193–208
post-capitalist power 206
post-structuralism 22, 180
power(s) 54, 57, 59, 87, 200; of becom-
    ing 59; centrifugal 173; diagnostic 80;
    external 201–202, 203; and images
    68, 69, 72, 176; of language 109; of
    markets 13, 204, 206–207; in matter
    106, 109; non-personal 85, 87; outside
    space and time 175; patrician 198;

post-capitalist 206; procreative 86; ruling 115; of the soul 177, 182; of the spirit 182; transcendent 201–202, 203; and the truth 196; unequal 196; of the virtual 40; weaving 178; will to 87, 188n40; of the world 179
power law distribution 132
pre-existent wholes 10, 29, 30–31, 32, 36, 37, 41, 42
primordial nature, of the divine 40
private thinker 52, 64, 66, 69, 70, 74n16
Process and Reality 41
procreation 86
prognosis 102, 117
Prophetissa, Maria 11, 107, 111
Proust and Signs 4, 28
psyche, the 3, 12, 13, 52, 69, 96, 140; and archetypes 105, 114; and dispersal 139; and edusemiotic self 103, 117, 122; and holism 23, 33; invisible elements of 120; of modern man 53, 60; plasticity of 98; self-regulation of 85–86; and shadow 115; and similarity 179–180; structural elements of; and symbol 132; and wholeness 135
psychic fragmentation 3
psychic reality 7, 33
psychic wholeness 12, 32, 67, 88, 139
psychoanalysis 5, 6, 11, 51, 81, 82, 84, 97, 98
psychoanalytic literary criticism 83–84
psychoid archetype 7, 26
Psychological Achievements of Friedrich Nietzsche, The 175
psychological concepts 140
psychological development 22–23
psychological education 67, 69
psychological healing 22–23
psychological model, of Jung 3, 10, 26, 35
psychological wholeness 3, 23, 24
psychology, depth 43, 51, 104, 105
psychopathology 84
psychophysical correlations 143, 144, 149, 157–158
psychophysical unity 139
psychophysically neutral reality 12, 13; and exceptional experiences 143, 144, 146, 150, 151, 153, 154–155, 158, 159

psychotherapy 3, 8, 23, 90, 91–92, 94, 98
pure immanence 4, 10, 33–34, 38, 40, 44, 109

quadratic form 125, 126, 127, 135, 139
quantum nonlocality *145*
quantum physics 68, 144, 146
quaternity 107, 135, 138, 139–140, 151

rational agent 118
rationalistic Weltanschauung 53, 55, 58, 63–64, 74n17
rationality 26, 93–94, 105; *see also* irrationality
realism, local 146–148
reality: of appearance 177; background 150; epistemic levels of 144–145; holistic 145, 147; of images 13, 176–178, 188n42; of life 178; local 147; models of 155; ontic levels of 144–145, 147, 154; physical 23, 111; psychic 7, 33; self-model of 155, 157; transcendental 32; unitary 8; world-model of 155, 157
reason 26, 63, 64, 110, 116, 196
rebirth 75n25, 115, 116
reciprocal determination 39
recognition 66, 67, 68, 69
reconciliation 2, 3, 26, 112
recursion 130, 133
Red Book, The 3, 91, 93, 94, 98, 184–185
reductionism 2
reification/reified experiences 9, 13, 157, 158, 159, 160, 163n12
relational entities 102
relational experiences 13, 157, 158, 160
relations: bidirectional 149, 154; of exteriority 7, 52, 57–58; external 30, 41; internal 7, 30–32; social 6, 95
religion 51, 55, 56, 66, 68, 181; of contingency 194, 207; and holism 26, 27, 42; and symptomatology 82, 94–95, 97
representations 9, 32, 63, 69, 91, 92, 125–126, 172; and edusemiotic self 106, 113, 120; and exceptional experiences 152, 153, 155, 158
resistance 30, 58, 59, 68, 71, 118
restored wholes 10, 29, 30–31, 32, 36, 37, 41, 42

rhizome 7, 80, 81, 97, 98, 108–109,
    116–117; *see also* image of thought
River Map, The *130*
Royal science 56
ruling powers 115

sadism/sado-masochism 80
scaling 131–132, 133
schizoanalysis 106
secret immanence, of the divine
    spirit 106
Seele 13, 174, 175, 179; *see also* soul
self, the 3, 10, 12, 62, 64–65, 89, 104,
    128; and exceptional experiences
    150–151, 160; and holism 22–23,
    24–25, 32, 36, 37–38, 42–43, 44–45n4
self-education 11, 103–104, 120–121, *121*
self-knowledge 11, 104
self-model, of reality 155, 157
self-reflection 121
self-similarity 132
self-transcendence 122
semiotics 102–122, *108*, *121*, 121
sensible objects 33, 119
shadow archetype 12, 24–25, 32, 150,
    160; and edusemiotic self 115–116,
    117–118, 119, 122
shared collectivity 25
signs 6, 9, 11, 82, 83, 179–180, 198; and
    edusemiotic self 102–122
similarity 13, 132, 171–172, 176, 178,
    179, 181–182; elementary 13, 177–178,
    179–180
Simpson, Christopher 39
Smuts, Jan Christiaan 2, 3, 20, 21, 44n3
social entities 23, 44n2
social life 193, 195, 196, 197, 200, 201,
    203, 207n8
social order 68, 76n27, 193, 194,
    195–196, 202, 205
social relations 6, 95
social valorization 204
socialism 54, 196
society 1, 24, 56, 60, 68, 72n3, 118; and
    markets 195, 197, 198, 200, 202, 205
Socratism 175
soul 13, 69, 87, 92, 110, 153, 160; and
    holistic enchantment and eternal

recurrence 174, 175, 176, 177, 179,
    180, 182
space 57–58, 88, 114, 120, 122, 160–161,
    175, 178
Spinoza, Baruch 5, 143, 167, 172, 196;
    and exceptional experiences 144, 153,
    161–162n1; and holism 34, 42,
    45n5
spirit 2, 23, 81, 106, 109, 119, 158, 160;
    and eternal recurrence 168, 174, 175,
    179, 180, 182
Spirit as Adversary of the Soul, The 174,
    175, 179
spirituality 7, 20, 118
State, the 52–59, 61, 63, 65,
    69, 71
State-form 52–59
State-religion 53
State-science 53
State-thinker 71
static representations 9, 106
static transcendence 41
statistical levelling down 53
statistical man 11, 51, 53, 64
Steiner, Rudolf 168
striated space 58
structural correlations 154–155
structuralism 180
subject, dissolution of the 65, 90
subjective consciousness 149–150
submission, to market laws 196
substance 5, 74n18, 109, 143
superordinate totality 32
symbolic density 132
symbolic structures 132
symbolic world, of psychic
    wholeness 139
symbolism 126–127, 140
symbols 9, 11, 12, 89, 177, 179, 180; and
    edusemiotic self 102, 109, 114; and
    holism 23, 26, 37–38; and wholeness
    132, 135, 138
symptomatology 80–98
symptoms 9, 11, 82–83, 94, 102–103,
    116, 117
synchronicity 7, 12, 111, 112, 140,
    151–155, 157–158; and holism 26–27,
    31, 32, 33, 38

synthesis: from analysis to 119–122, *121*; of conscious and unconscious 37, 42–43

Tarot, as a sign-system 119–121, *121*, 121–122
temple dream 96–97
tertium non datur 105, 107
tertium quid 11, 105, 111, 150
theism 7, 10, 32–42, 45n5, 45n6, 45n7, 74n20
therapeutics 82
therapy 3, 20, 82, 87, 90; *see also* psychotherapy
thought: Eastern 9; habits of 60; holistic 2–3, 7, 9, 20, 21–30, 36, 42; image of 11, 51, 52, 60–71; mystical 7, 9; outside 70, 71; systems of 10, 51; totalitarian 8, 33, 42
Thousand Plateaus: Capitalism and Schizophrenia, A 52, 54, 59, 60, 65
Thus Spoke Zarathustra 13, 169–170, 183
time 88, 114, 122, 160–161, 175
total personality *see* totality
totalitarian intuitions 3
totalitarian regimes 54
totalitarian thought 8, 33, 42
totalitarianism 20–21, 42
totality: Deleuze on 10, 28–29, 73n10, 86, 122; Jung on 52, 138; Nietzsche's view of Goethe on 167; Pauli on 148; peripheral 86; superordinate 32
totalization 30
transcendence 4, 10, 106, 109, 122, 157–161; and holism 22, 26, 29–44
transcendent power 201–202, 203
transcendental empiricism 113
transcendental field 109, 111, 114
transcendental reality 32
transcendental unconscious 106
transdisciplinarity 1–2
transformation 24, 62, 66, 109
Transformation and Symbols of the Libido/Symbols of Transformation 184–185
transgressivity 86, 109, 158, 160
transversal communication 109
transversal holism 7

true life 108–109
Twilight of the Idols 167
typical reality models 12

Übermensch 170, 183
ultimate wholeness 8, 14
uncertainty 13, 32, 81, 117, 193, 201, 207
unconscious, the 3, 5–6, 9, 11, 68, 75n25, 128, 135; autonomous 91, 98; collective *see* collective unconscious; and edusemiotic self 102–122; and exceptional experiences 144, 146, 148–150, 154, 160; and holism 23, 26, 35, 39, 43; objective 149–150; and symptomatology 86–87, 88, 90, 91, 92, 97; transcendental 106
unconscious shadow 115
underground man 63
undiscovered self (present and future), The 10, 42, 51–76
unequal power 196
unidirectional correlations 154
unio mentalis 23–24, 160
union of opposites 22–23, 135, 158
union of the conscious and unconscious personality 22–23
unitary reality 8
unities 135, 138
unity of opposites 22–23, 135, 158
unity of the self 12
universal interconnectedness, among all aspects of reality 26
univocity of being 4
unus mundus 3, 10, 12, 106, 112; and archetypes 150–151; and exceptional experiences *145*, 153, 160, 161; and holism 23, 26–27, 31, 32, 37; and symmetries 162n6

value: dimension of 116–117; in Jung's psychological model 26; market-based 199, 201, 203
vertigo, games of 201, 202
vertigo of philosophy 163n10; *see also* immanence
violence 116
virtual, the 4, 39, 40–41, 111–112, 114, 120, 162n3

virtual archetypes 12
vision (in Jungian analysis) 104–105
vision (sight) 11, 65, 84, 90, 91, 98
visions (dreams) 24, 92, 95, 110, 176
vitalisms 7, 61, 87, 116

war machines 58, 70, 73n12
wealth inequality 207n8
weaving power, of all that belongs
    together through relation or
    opposition 178
Weltanschauung 53, 55, 58, 61,
    63–64, 74n17
What is Philosophy? 4, 62
Whitehead, Alfred North 21, 40–41, 44,
    161–162n1
whole, the: bounded 65; integrated
    112–113; open 4, 8, 32–33; symbolic
    knowledge of 8
whole man 11, 51–52, 58, 59, 62, 63,
    66, 69, 71

wholeness: archetype of 31, 89, 103, 104;
    geometry of 125–140, *126*, *127*, *128*,
    129, *130*, *131*, *134*, *135*, *136*, *137*, *138*;
    of humanity 22, 24; psychic 12, 32,
    67, 88, 139; psychological 3, 23, 24;
    ultimate 8, 14
wholes 1–2, 9, 10, 144, 152; and holism
    24, 28, 29, 30–31, 32, 36, 37, 41, 42
Will to Power, The (book) 176
will to power (concept) 87, 188n40
woman's dream, Mandala based
    on a *131*
world-model, of reality 155, 157
wounded healer 89–90

Zarathustra 13, 168, 169–171, 173,
    183
Zipf, George Kingsly/Zipf's law
    132, 133
Zofingia Lectures 73n6, 74n19
Zofingiaverein 59, 74n14

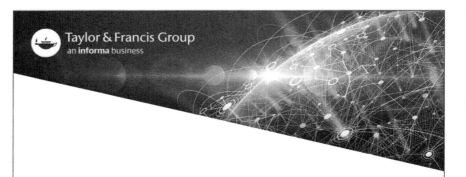